PRISONERS
WITHOUT
BARS

a caregiver's tale

donna o'donnell figurski

Virginia

Published in the United States by WriteLife Publishing
(An imprint of Boutique of Quality Books Publishing Company)
www.writelife.com

978-1-60808-205-6 (p)
978-1-60808-206-3 (e)

Library of Congress Control Number: 2018956542

Book design by Robin Krauss, www.bookformatters.com
Cover design by Marla Thompson, www.edgeofwater.com

First editor: Olivia Swenson
Second editor: Caleb Guard

To my best friend and husband, David—not only a survivor of traumatic brain injury, but also a conqueror. Your road back from the other side was an arduous one, yet you executed each step with grace and poise. You are as amazing as you were on the first day I met you. There was magic then. There still is. Thank you for staying with me. Of course, you know I would never have forgiven you if you had left me too soon. I love you—always will. Three squeezes!

CONTENTS

FOREWORD

David and Donna's story is one of the tragic possibilities that life affords us. We must exercise our abilities to their fullest extent to make the best of our most challenging trials. This is exemplified not only by Donna's family trauma, but also by their progressive and heartfelt triumph. Donna's narrative explains traumatic brain injury and its multiple destructive tentacles, while showing us the power of love, dedication, and persistence.

I admire and respect David and Donna's battle to overcome what so many of us cannot imagine. They have reintroduced us to the meaning of our existence and to the sanctity of its preservation.

This account has reinforced my dedication to my profession. Medicine for me has always been a unique privilege to heal and comfort. A physician's knowledge and training must provide thorough and evidence-based competence, but always with compassion and professionalism. Every day, I am reminded of my oath to serve as a healer by being a trusted liaison between formidable illness and human beings.

David and Donna have my admiration, and I thank them for allowing me to assist in their quest to overcome incredible adversity.

Michael Kailas, MD
Neurologist
New Jersey

PREFACE

When my husband, David, suffered what the neurosurgeons called a traumatic brain injury (TBI) in January of 2005, his world was upended. Mine was redesigned. I never intended to write his story. My expertise lies in writing for children, not adults. Besides, I had no time. I barely survived each day as I took up residence in whichever of the three hospitals David was a "guest." Writing this book never crossed my mind.

But I did write. I wrote wordy informational emails to family and friends across the country, explaining each minute detail of David's day. I called the emails "updates." They were my lifelines to folks outside my immediate world. Until I began work on this book a year later in 2006, I didn't realize how crucial those emails were, as were the digital recordings I scrupulously kept each time I spoke with a doctor, nurse, or therapist. Without these histories, I would've had to rely on sketchy memories.

Though I made no conscious effort to write this book, words flowed late each night, after I put David to bed and when my defenses were fragile. That is when I cried. Releasing suppressed emotions and tears allowed me to face each new day. In this way, David's story unfolded, and I realized I had to tell it. I expect that the writing of this book, memories stumbling across my mind and words spilling onto the screen, was therapeutic.

David emerged on the other side of TBI, though he didn't arrive unscathed. Neither of us had. He had, and still has, many obstacles to overcome, but David's story is how one man survived and is conquering traumatic brain injury with patience, persistence, and grace. He is an inspiration not only to family and friends, but also to everyone he meets—and especially to me, who lives his daily struggle.

My sincere wish is that survivors of traumatic brain injury can identify with and relate to David's story and gain solace from it. I hope those with TBI—either through closed-brain injuries like David's, or from an unfortunate accident or from the ravages of war (many of our returning soldiers are afflicted with TBI)—know that they are not alone. I feel for their caregivers, and I want to offer them my encouragement. I hope that David's story will inspire other survivors as Jill Bolte Taylor's book, *My Stroke of Insight: A Brain Scientist's Personal Journey*; Lee and Bob Woodruff's book, *In an Instant: A Family's Journey of Love and Healing*; Gabrielle Giffords and Mark Kelly's book, *Gabby: A Story of Courage, Love and Resilience*; and Rosemary Rawlins' book, *Learning by Accident: A Caregiver's True Story of Fear, Family, and Hope*, inspired both David and me. Finally, I hope that *Prisoners without Bars: A Caregiver's Tale* will provide a thread of hope to all and offer a slice of a new life after TBI.

Donna O'Donnell Figurski
Arizona

PROLOGUE

Before David 's traumatic brain injury, we lived a normal life. We both grew up in Erie, Pennsylvania. I went to a girls' high school; he went to the boys' school. I lived on the west side of town, while he lived on the east side. On that starry night in 1965 when I met him, I knew he would be my life partner. He didn't know it yet. He knew by 1969, when we said our vows. I was twenty and he was twenty-two.

We lived a normal life. David finished college and went on to graduate school. I went to cosmetology school at night and cared for our daughter during the day. We moved from Pittsburgh, Pennsylvania, to Rochester, New York, to San Diego, California, to Tenafly, New Jersey, adding another child, our son, along the way.

We lived a normal life as David went from assistant professor to full professor at Columbia University, and I earned my teaching certification from William Paterson University. I then taught first or third grade at Honiss School in Dumont, New Jersey, the town in which we raised our children.

We lived a normal life as we watched our children grow. We spent our time at gymnastic studios, soccer fields, cross-country courses, and softball fields. We went to parent-teacher conferences and back-to-school nights. We watched proudly as both children graduated college and took up their own lives.

We lived a normal life as empty nesters in New Jersey. We continued our date nights on Friday and Saturday, and sometimes, for extra measure, we had one mid-week too. We both enjoyed our jobs, and life was good.

We lived a normal life until the dawn of January 13, 2005. Then we didn't.

CHAPTER 1

Everything's Blurry

Each morning, David slipped from bed at 4:00 a.m.—quietly, so as not to wake me. He went to his home office across the hall and spent forty minutes in a series of exercises. He put on his headset and listened to "Sun Spirit" by Deuter or Chinese bamboo flute music as he performed his version of tai chi. It was his way of getting ready for the day. Then he showered, did a few chin-ups, and got dressed. Before he left for his lab, he would creep into our bedroom and leave a kiss on my cheek. Sometimes I pretended to be asleep. Sometimes I sleepily waved goodbye. Other times I pulled him down for just one more "real" kiss before he left. Then I would roll over, pull up the blankets, and wait for my alarm to ring at 5:50 a.m. It was his schedule, and it was mine.

Ever since 9/11, when overwhelming traffic into New York City turned a thirty-minute commute into a one- to two-hour nightmare, David began this unrealistic schedule. Rising early to beat the morning traffic and not returning home until well after rush hour—7:00 or 8:00 p.m.—was a very long day.

On January 13, 2005, David's morning started much the same as it did each day. The only difference was that he delayed his rising by one hour. He planned to work at home that morning, preparing a talk about his research that he expected to deliver at Wesleyan University in Connecticut on Saturday. A long-time professor-friend was retiring from the faculty, and David was a featured speaker at his retirement symposium. It was an invitation and an honor that may have saved David's life.

If David's morning had been routine, he would have been in his laboratory at Columbia University in New York City by 6:00 a.m.—long before his students arrived. If the morning had been routine, he would have been at his computer returning email, poring over recently collected data, and conducting business in his office, a beautiful room flanked by his two laboratories overlooking the George Washington Bridge on Manhattan's Upper West Side. If the morning had been routine, I wouldn't be writing this story. The morning was not routine, and that is why David lived through January 13th.

I was dressed and had applied the finishing touches to my makeup—"Brush and apply," as my friend Danielle always teased me. I looked at the clock. It was 7:00 a.m. *I'm okay*, I thought. If I left by 7:20 a.m., I could make it to school with plenty of time to prepare. The children arrived at 8:40 a.m. I used to live in the same town where I taught first and third grade on alternate years. It was a roll-out-of-bed commute— only five minutes from school. So easy! But in 2001, David and I moved to a new home in a community fifty minutes away.

I loved our new home, but I was not crazy about my commute. Half of it was highway driving, and the traffic could be unpredictable in the City area. A fifty-minute, no-traffic commute could take just that, or it could take up to ninety minutes. I always left extra time for snarls or accidents. Throw in an early morning Pupil Assistance Committee meeting or a parent-teacher conference, and I had to leave even earlier. Thursday, January 13, 2005, started out as a relatively normal day. I planned to leave by 7:20 a.m. But I didn't.

Just after 7:00 a.m., David stumbled into our bedroom. His hand covered his right eye. "I can't see!" he cried, panic in his voice. "Everything's blurry!"

Pain etched his face as he collapsed on the bed. When he removed his hand, his right eye was filled with blood. He told me he had been doing chin-ups. He did thirteen of them—one more than he had done the day before. That's David—always pushing, trying to surpass his last accomplished goal, only to surpass that achievement the next time. I remember thinking, *Why? Why did you have to do one more? Why wasn't twelve enough? Or ten or even five?* But it wasn't enough. It never was.

I wanted to call the paramedics. I had the phone in my hand. It was like a lifeline, but David refused to let me call. He wanted to wait a few more minutes to see if his pain subsided. He sat at the edge of the bed, continuing to cover his eye. Soon the pain spread. I told him to tell me what was happening in case I had to tell a doctor. The pain spread down his cheek, then through his forehead. As it intensified, it moved quickly to the back of his head, and I would wait no longer. He agreed. I dialed 9-1-1.

The dispatcher sounded bored. I guess after hearing emergency calls day and night, the essence of emergency wears off, and anyhow, it wasn't *her* emergency. It wasn't *her* husband who was suffering. To me, the call was surreal. It seemed to be matter-of-fact, business-as-usual for her. "What is the nature of your emergency?" she asked (sip of coffee). "What is your address?" (bite of bagel). If we had been talking about the weather, there would have been more emotion.

"Can you believe it's been raining for two weeks?"

"I know! Make it stop!"

The dispatcher showed no emotion, and my emotion soared off the scale. It would have been helpful if she had shown some compassion, even pretended to understand the crisis David and I were trapped in.

Dictionary.com defines "emergency" as "a sudden, urgent, usually unexpected occurrence or occasion requiring immediate action." I wanted immediate action, but the paramedics were not magically at the door as soon as I dropped the receiver into the cradle. I wrapped my arms around David, who was writhing and groaning in pain on the bed.

"They're coming, David. They're coming. Everything's going to be all right. Just hang on, David. I love you so much. I love you. I love you!" I spouted this litany like a broken record.

If love or words could have made a difference, the emergency would have ended immediately. Love was not enough, and it didn't end. David kept saying variations of "Donna, I love you. My life has been good. We've had a good life. I love you!" And he added, "Tell the kids I love them too . . . and Treska and Kaya. Everything you need is in the file. The papers are in the file." The papers! I didn't want to hear about papers. That was too serious. The papers meant only one thing: David didn't think he would come home again. I couldn't let my mind go there. I wouldn't listen. I had a general idea of where the papers were, but I wanted nothing to do with them.

"David, I don't need the papers! Don't worry about that. Everything's going to be okay. I love you!"

Where were the paramedics? I ran to the window. No sign of them. Panic struck me—I had forgotten to give the dispatcher the gate code. It was too early for the guard to be on duty. How would they get in? I dialed 9-1-1 again. Same dispatcher. (I hope she finished her bagel.)

"Sorry to interrupt again, but I forgot to tell you the code to the gate." I rattled off the numbers. It didn't occur to me that emergency vehicles would have access to the code at the gate. But they surely didn't have access to my front door, and it was locked. I ran down two sets of stairs in our brownstone-like townhouse. Slipping and sliding would be a better description, as I took the stairs two at a time. When I nearly tripped on the first staircase, I realized I had better slow down. I would be no help to David with a twisted ankle, but I needed to get to the door. I wanted to leave the door open, so the paramedics could rush in and take charge.

By the time I got back upstairs, David writhed on the bed, moaning, and sweat poured from his body. I could do nothing but rub his arm and try to comfort and reassure him that everything was going to be all right. But I didn't believe it. I had never been so scared. Though he was the one in physical danger and pain, I saw my life draining away. We had lived a normal life, and now we were sharing a tragedy.

CHAPTER 2

Paramedics Don't Always Rush

Finally, the ambulance arrived. I dashed again to the door to guide the paramedics to the bedroom. I expected them to rush. Instead, they slowly ambled around their truck to gather their equipment. Then they slowly climbed the stairs to the bedroom. They asked David what was bothering him. David attempted to speak, but his words tumbled over each other. He was nearly unintelligible. Maybe he should have said, "Oh geez, I have a headache!"

These guys must be related to the dispatcher, I thought. I wondered why they didn't comprehend the urgency. David continued to writhe and moan as I recounted the details—the thirteen chin-ups, something bursting in David's head, the rapid spread of pain. When one member of the crew finally placed an oxygen mask over David's face, relief came. David became silent, and I was grateful. He looked peaceful. I later realized that David had slipped into a coma. That was bad, but at least for the moment, it brought him peace.

The paramedics strapped David to a gurney, securing him for the trip down the stairs. It was a good thing too, because they bounced him and the gurney off of our newly painted walls—black smudges on Sugar Cookie in the hallways and black splotches on Suntan Yellow in the foyer. Later, I tried to scrub away these reminders of this unpleasant memory, but they could not be erased. Dabs of paint would cover them in time, but my memory of that morning would never be erased.

"Which hospital do you want to go to?" one paramedic asked me.

"Columbia-Presbyterian," I quickly answered. "David works at Columbia. It's where he will want to be."

"Sorry," he said. "We don't go to the City."

"But that's always been our hospital of choice."

"Can't cross the George Washington Bridge. It's out of our jurisdiction," he told me. "Sorry."

I didn't know what to do. I didn't know any hospitals here. We had moved to the area a few years ago, and hospitals were not on our minds. I guess we should have thought of it. We should have had a plan, but we didn't. I asked the paramedics to suggest a good hospital. They skirted my question, as if they knew there were good hospitals and ones not so good, but they refused to recommend one. That was likely protocol, and I understood their need to remain impartial, but it did not seem fair. This was life or death, and the right hospital could make the difference. I am sure, with all of their transports, they knew the best hospitals.

Since they would not suggest one, I asked which hospitals were nearby. A paramedic suggested several. Two were fifteen minutes away. At least now I had a choice—Sierta Hospital or Blum Hospital. I had never heard of Blum, but I had passed Sierta while running errands. Though I never paid it much mind, at least it sounded familiar. We went to Sierta.

The paramedics loaded David into the back of the ambulance. David tells me now that he vaguely remembers being jostled in, but he remembers nothing after that. I wanted to ride in the back with David, but the driver firmly suggested I sit up front. Though he did not say anything, I could discern the seriousness on his face. I realized I would only be in the way. I debated following in my own car. When I asked the paramedics if they could return me home after David was through, their incredulous expressions helped me realize how out of it I was. It was my first experience riding in an ambulance. I had no idea when I left my home that morning that it would be days before I returned.

As I rode in the front, I could not see what was happening in the back, but I could hear. It didn't sound good. About a mile from our home the ambulance pulled to the curb, near Dunkin' Donuts. *What's happening? Why are they stopping? We are supposed to be rushing to the hospital. This is an emergency!* These thoughts rambled through my head. The driver told me not to get out. I did not. I was too scared. Another ambulance pulled up behind us, and another crew hopped aboard. We were off again.

They began to work on David. I don't know what they were doing, but one attendant kept yelling at the driver to go more slowly. More slowly? We were only going twenty miles per hour. I wanted to go eighty, a hundred, but even at twenty, every bump seemed like being dropped from a cliff. I thought that an ambulance would provide a soft, gentle ride—like riding in a limousine. Not true! It was more like being pulled down a dirt road in a rickety red wagon. *How can this be good for an injured person?* Slowly, slowly we continued our "fifteen-minute" journey to the hospital, which took more than double that time.

When I finally saw the hospital, I breathed more easily. *Now everything will be all right,* I thought. *The emergency doctors and nurses will make David better.* The ambulance stopped at the emergency entrance. I hopped out and went to the back of the truck. The doors did not open. I sensed movement and heard voices inside, though they were indiscernible. What was taking them so long? Hurry! Another ambulance pulled up. I wanted David's ambulance doors to fly open, and I wanted the paramedics to rush him into the emergency room. I did not want some other emergency to go ahead of him. What if there was only one doctor? What if this were like the deli, and we had to take a number?

I paced, and I waited, and my mind screamed. I could do nothing . . . but wait. I would be perfecting my skill of waiting over the next few years. Finally, the doors to the ambulance opened, and I sighed in relief. I saw David on the gurney, his eyes closed, not moving. I looked for the rise and fall of his chest. The blanket moved slightly, but it *did* move. Then the legs on the gurney dropped down, and David was pushed through the doors marked "Emergency."

CHAPTER 3

No. I Mean, Yes

The paramedics pushed David down the short hall into a little cubicle, an examining room. They moved him from the gurney to the observation bed. The doctor and nurses quickly took over. They did not pull the privacy curtain closed, and though I was surprised, I was grateful. I did not want to be separated from David. I needed to know what was happening.

I watched from the reception desk, where I had to produce my insurance card. I hoped it was in my wallet. I rarely used it. It is the kind of thing you put there and forget about. I found it and handed it to Janis, the receptionist. She did not seem particularly friendly or compassionate—what you would expect from someone in this position, who sees emergencies and distraught people every day. She was business-like, just doing her job.

She handed me a clipboard. I sighed as I glanced at the numerous forms and endless questions. This was the beginning of the paperwork, which would stalk me throughout this journey. When I completed the forms and returned them to her, she had even more questions. But she probably got more than she asked for.

Janis asked if I had called my family. I shook my head no. I said I had a cousin who lived down the street from me, but she was in Florida visiting her parents. Her husband, who had remained home, was working in the City, and I didn't want to bother him. I had another cousin who lived about a half hour from the hospital, but she and her husband were also working. They were not an option either. I explained that we were all from the Pittsburgh area and that we had all moved here at different times. Essentially there was no one to call. I told her that the next nearest relative was David's father, who lived in Erie, about 450 miles away. There was no point in calling. I did not want to scare him. I would tell him when this was over . . . when everything was better. I could handle this. Sure I could! I bit my lip to hold back the tears.

I would not cry. I needed to feel in control. I didn't want to break down. I could not take the chance of David seeing my tears or sensing my anxiety. I believe that, although a person is unconscious or in a coma, he or she is aware at some level. My desire to convey confidence may have made me seem cavalier, but I wanted David, if he was aware, to feel that all would be fine. It *was* going to be fine! It had to be. I was being stoic for him and probably more for me. I knew if I cried, if I broke down and lost control, then I was accepting defeat. I would be admitting that there was a serious problem, and I was not willing to accept that. I would be unable to do what I needed to unless I stayed strong. I would do whatever it took.

Completing the paperwork and my discussion with Janis probably took three times longer than it would have if I hadn't been stealing glances toward the examining room. My mind was not on the paperwork. When I finished, I went into the examining room—right up to the head of the bed. I held David's hand, and my litany started again. "I love you. Everything's going to be all right, David. I love you."

The doctors and nurses were patient with me. They welcomed

me. Nina was the nurse in charge of David in the emergency room. She was gentle and seemed genuinely concerned. I wanted to hug her. The cubicle was small with machines and cabinets pushed against the wall, and yet Nina and Dr. Faber worked around me. I soon realized that I was in the way, and my selfish need to be with my husband could impede their efforts to make him better. I told them I would wait outside. Nina declined my offer and pointed to a chair along the wall. Still they crawled over me. They continued their examination, probing and sticking David with needles and attaching tubes and questioning me. I recounted what I had already told the paramedics and what I would be retelling repeatedly for the following weeks, even months, to various physicians, nurses, and therapists.

"David was exercising. He was doing chin-ups. He did thirteen of them, one more than he did the day before, and something burst inside his head."

After more probing by the doctor and what seemed to be endless assessment by Nina, she asked me if I had any children. When I nodded yes, she asked if I had called them.

"No," I said and shook my head. "Do you think I need to?"

"You should call them." She emphasized each word.

A wave of panic engulfed me, and I shook it off. An ostrich with her head in the sand—that was me, and that was how I wanted to be. If I pushed this reality away, if I did not believe this horror, then it could not really be happening. Could it?

Soon they rushed David upstairs for a CT (CAT, or computed tomography) scan. Nina said to wait in the waiting room and she would find me when they returned. I did not see a waiting room. I stood by the reception desk, looking like a pitiful soul or someone who had just lost her best friend. I guess both were true.

Janis, the receptionist, took pity on me. She again asked if there was anyone I could call to be with me. She too asked if I had any children.

"Could they come?"

"No," I replied. "I mean yes."

She looked confused, and I did not blame her. I was not making sense, and I tried to clarify. "They live a world away. My son lives in California, and my daughter lives in New Mexico. I don't want them to worry. Besides, they are busy in their lives."

Janis was surprised to learn that I had children that old. She wanted to know more. Perhaps this was her way of distracting me from the present trauma. It did not, but it did make waiting for David to return from the CT scan more bearable.

I told her that my son, Jared, graduated from the University of California at Santa Cruz (UCSC) with a degree in marine biology. He worked at the university after graduation and was now doing his graduate work to earn his PhD in the same field. I told her that, as a child, Jared voraciously read every fish magazine he could find. His bedroom was filled with aquariums and fish equipment. I smiled as I remembered how Jared invented a device, using tubing and a plastic liter bottle, to separate brine shrimp hatchlings from their eggshells. I prattled on about how Jared got hooked on marine biology when he caught his first fish on a string and a paperclip in the stream behind my father's house in Fairview, Pennsylvania. Jared was only four years old.

With my mind alert for David's return, I continued to chatter distractedly. I told Janis story after story. If I had not been surrounded with white-frocked doctors rushing by, the incessant buzzing of various monitors, and the occasional code alert from the PA system, I could almost imagine I was socializing at an afternoon tea. It was a good distraction, and Janis was a good listener.

I told her how Jared had worked at the Maria Mitchell Aquarium on Nantucket during his high school summers. He went out in the Zodiac, an inflatable boat with an outboard motor, to collect samples from the ocean. He set up aquariums to display his treasures. He conducted tours and taught youngsters and their parents about underwater life. I also explained that Jared was a diver and had been the captain of the *Paragon*, the university's thirty-two-foot research vessel, before beginning his graduate research. I told Janis that I would call Jared later, if it became necessary.

I then rambled on about my daughter, Kiersten. She had gone to Bard College, an impressive school. The student-professor ratio is 10:1, and students are encouraged to design their own curricula. I explained how a group of students wanted to learn German, and a course was established to immerse them in the language. After two intense terms, they went to Germany to study at Heidelberg University. I explained that Kiersten had become fluent and returned to Germany after she graduated. When Kiersten was living with friends in Regensburg, she met her husband-to-be, Falko, and they moved to Leipzig, where they became the parents of two lovely daughters, Treska and Kaya. Kiersten taught English as a second language there, but after the birth of her daughters, she desperately wanted to be a midwife. Though her initial plan was to train in Germany, where she had lived for nearly eight years, research on the web brought her to the Northern New Mexico Women's Health and Birth Center and the National College of Midwifery.

After three days of rigorous interviews, Kiersten was chosen as one of two students accepted into the program. She was overjoyed. Kiersten, Falko, and the girls moved to the States. I was happy too, expecting that they would be easier to visit now that we were all on the same continent. Not true! It usually took about fifteen hours to get to Leipzig door-to-door. With a three-hour drive from the airport in Albuquerque to their home in Taos, it took about the same time. I was not inclined to call her to make that long trip. I could handle this. I told Janis that I would call Kiersten later, if it became necessary.

As I spilled bits and pieces of my life, Janis lost her business-as-usual demeanor and invited me to sit with her behind the reception desk. I guessed she did not want me to be alone. I did not want to be alone either. Not ever! I babbled on. I told her that David was a professor of microbiology at Columbia University and that he was the healthiest person I knew. He was fanatic about taking care of himself, eating well, and exercising. David even put vitamins on the counter for me each morning.

"He shouldn't be here," I said. "What went wrong?"

I also told her how lucky we were because neither of us had left for work. I told her that he was my best friend and I could not lose him. I held back my tears, but I think a few seeped out anyway. I told her how David and I met at a dance when I was only sixteen, and how I told my mother that I would marry him someday. I knew! Just as I knew he had to get better. He was my whole life. I rambled on, and Janis listened as I waited.

CHAPTER 4

Unthinkable Odds

A doctor rushed in. He seemed to be looking for someone. Me, I guessed, but since I was behind the reception counter, he seemed confused. When he noticed me and recovered, he thrust his hand into mine.

"I'm Dr. Hulda," he said. "Your husband is in very good shape."

Relief washed over me, until—

"He'll make a good organ donor."

"What?!" I shook my head. My body began to tremble. I wanted to shout, "*No! No!* You're supposed to save him. He's *not* going to be an organ donor!" But I stood planted. More thoughts whirred through my brain. I vaguely remembered David telling me that he intended to be a donor. I knew there was a section on the New Jersey driver's license where one could check organs to donate—eyes, kidney, heart, liver, etc. I had not opted to be a donor, but I knew David had. I was secretly relieved I had forgotten his wallet. It was safe at home on his desk.

Thinking fast, I managed to say, "Uhh, I don't believe he chose that." I knew donating organs was an unselfish and honorable act. If I or someone I cared about were in need, I would be grateful to a donor, but I couldn't stop the ungenerous thoughts. Perhaps the doctor's eagerness raised a red flag. I wondered if he had someone waiting for a set of eyes or a heart. David's heart? No! That belonged to me. I wondered if the doctor would fight as hard to save David's life if he had another patient in the wings who would benefit from David's organs.

I again proclaimed, "David didn't want that." I wonder now, if I had not insisted, would David's eyes be looking out of someone else's body? Would his heart beat for a new love? I do not regret my white lie.

Dr. Hulda told me that he had seen David's CT scan on his home computer and came immediately. He explained that David had suffered a cerebellar hemorrhage. Blood was filling his brain and causing intense pressure. The pressure needed to be released to minimize the damage. Dr. Hulda laid out options for me, and none was desirable. He said that another CT scan could determine if the pressure was easing, but it would waste valuable time if it were not. Another option was immediate surgery.

I must have looked like a zombie. I stood mute, wringing my hands, breathing out and in and out again. I didn't know what to do. I felt paralyzed. My permission was needed to operate on my husband's brain. How could I give it? How could I allow Dr. Hulda to work on my husband's beautiful, smart brain?

Dr. Hulda watched my pain and indecision and said, "Come. Let me show you." I followed him to an office around the corner. With a few quick taps of his fingers, the computer screen lit up with what looked like a skull. Dr. Hulda outlined the dark section and explained it was blood filling David's skull.

I stared. *This can't be happening*, I thought. *How can this be real?* I felt trapped in a science fiction movie. Brain surgery! I tried to focus. My brain felt like the one I was gaping at on the screen—completely useless. Again Dr. Hulda outlined my options and gave me survival percentages. He said we could gamble and do another CT scan. If the pressure had diminished—good. However, if it had not and was becoming more intense, then David would have a one in six hundred chance of living. *Unthinkable odds*, I thought. He went on to say that if David went immediately to surgery, his possibility of survival was better—one in twenty.

Still unthinkable! I stood there, panicky. How could I sign on the dotted line? What if I signed and David died on the table? What if I did not sign and he died anyway? I was in a no-win situation. I signed.

"Go!" I said. "Do the operation." I called after him, "Remember, he's my best friend in all the world."

Dr. Hulda canceled the CT scan and sent David directly to the operating room. I watched as Dr. Hulda dashed off to scrub. Soon he would open my husband's skull.

I vaguely remember following the attendant who pushed David's bed through the hospital corridors. He pushed David into a room with a large machine at its center. I watched through the wall-length window as the attendants, seemingly in slow motion, transferred David from his bed to a table. It didn't look like an operating room, at least not any I had seen in movies. I paced the length of the room, never taking my eyes off of David. Then the phone jangled, jarring me from my numbness. Though I was not able to hear the speaker, I knew something was wrong. I saw the nurse glance at David. Then like a bolt of lightning it struck me. This was the CT scan room!

"Oh no!" I nearly screamed. "Is that a CT scan machine?" Realizing it was, I did scream. "No! No! David's not supposed to be here. Dr. Hulda canceled the CT scan." The nurse looked confused. "We decided to go ahead with the surgery—immed- iately. He canceled the CT scan!" I repeated.

Now the nurses looked panicked. They quickly returned David to the bed, while assuring me that the operating room was just across the hall. I was not consoled. I fretted over time lost. As they pushed David through the operating room doors, I touched him—gently, as if I were afraid he would break. But he was already broken. I let him go with my love.

CHAPTER 5

Calling the World

The waiting room was small and nondescript. Chairs lined the walls, and there was a bathroom at one end. Like every hospital waiting room, it held the tears, the fears, and the memories of people in angst. I would leave three days and nights of my own angst to mix with the anxieties of those who came before me and those yet to come.

Three women were there, waiting for some relative or friend, I suppose. They were exchanging stories and laughing, and I guessed that their patient was here for a simple procedure—one that was not dangerous. I envied them. We did not exchange greetings, probably because I was centered on my grief. I couldn't see beyond myself or past my fears. I imagined what was happening behind those operating room doors, and it terrified me.

I brought a book with me. I had picked it up as I passed through my office before running down the steps and out my door to the ambulance. When did I think I would have time to read it? How did I think that I could concentrate? It was not like this was a routine doctor visit. We were going in an ambulance to an emergency room. But I always tote a book with me, and I recall feeling pleased that I remembered to grab it as I dashed out of the house. I also stuffed both David's and my cell phones and chargers into my backpack, and it was lucky that I did. They proved to be very valuable. I was charging phones all day.

I took Nina's advice and called my children. With the difference in time zones, it was early morning for both of them, and I hoped they would be awake. I imagined that Kiersten would soon be sending her daughters to school. It would be near 7:00 a.m. in Taos. Jared was probably rolling out of bed at 6:00 a.m. in Santa Cruz—expecting a normal, beautiful, new day on Monterey Bay. There would be no normal days for a long time, but we didn't know that yet. I was relieved when Kiersten and Jared both told me that they would catch the first available flight.

I imagined the flurry of calls between them and to the airlines to book flights. I knew Kiersten would have to make childcare arrangements for her daughters, Treska and Kaya. Jared would need to change his diving schedule and alert his advisor that he would be away indefinitely. This disruption of their lives is what I had hoped to avoid.

Next I called David's brothers, Tom and Pat, both in Detroit, and David's father, Hank, in Erie. A flurry of calls began there too. I didn't expect them to come, but come they did—Tom with his wife, Kathy, and Pat with his wife, Patrice. They are not only family, they are also close friends. I was grateful to have them with me for support, for counsel, and for company.

Then I called my mother in Phoenix, Arizona. She called my siblings, except for John. I called John and his wife, Carol, myself. It's near impossible to believe, but John and Carol were immersed in a similar nightmare with their twenty-four-year-old son. My nephew "Little" John suffered a traumatic brain injury three weeks earlier, just two days after Christmas. Little John was given a fifty percent chance of survival. Though he was no longer in critical danger, we were worried about him.

How could lightning strike twice in the same family? I needed to talk with John and Carol. I knew their pain. I had shared it with them for the past three weeks through phone calls and emails. I knew they would know mine.

I worried between the phone calls and between the thoughts of what was happening to David's brain on the operating table. I tried to excise the scary thoughts. They were hard to bear, and my imagination was working overtime. My mind raced ahead to every possibility. I didn't know then that this day was the beginning of a long worry phase in my life.

Earlier, when I was in the ambulance, I called my school secretary, Lillian, to explain what was happening to David and me. I told her I would not be in school that day, nor did I know when I would return. I asked her to hire a substitute for me. Lillian knew me well. She insisted that I not worry about school, but she knew I would. We had been friends since her daughter, Cathy, was in my third grade class many years ago.

Lillian also knew David well. They liked each other. I once convinced Lillian to go on a "date" with David many years ago while I was confined in a hospital. David and I had tickets to see the *Phantom of the Opera* on Broadway with my dad and my stepsister, who were visiting from Pennsylvania. I begged my doctor to allow me to go to the performance, but he refused, so I called Lil. She protested, but in vain. In the end, she went, and she loved the "date."

I called Lillian again while David was in surgery. I knew she'd offer words of encouragement to allay my fears. Lillian told me that my teaching assistant, Sheryl, was coming to be with me. I almost told Lillian to tell her not to come, but I stopped myself. I wanted Sheryl with me. We had a great working relationship. We talked and laughed and shared stories. I needed her support. She arrived soon after.

My cousin-in-law Bryce heard about David's crisis through the family grapevine. (Thank you, Alexander Graham Bell, for inventing the telephone, and Dr. Martin Cooper, for inventing the cell phone—both crucial communication devices during my crisis.) I did not know Bryce was coming, so I was surprised and relieved when he walked through the door. I valued his advice and was momentarily propped up and comforted by two close friends as we waited in the nondescript waiting room.

My phone continued to ring. I suppose that was good. Karen Bennett, the principal at Honiss School where I taught first grade, called to assure me that my class was fine. She insisted that I not worry about them and that she would take care of everything. Frankly, by this time I had stopped thinking about my first graders. My worries had escalated as David's brain underwent surgery.

Then I called Saul Silverstein, PhD, my magic man at Columbia. Saul was the chairman of the microbiology department, of which David was a member. He was also a friend. Saul's booming voice and take-charge manner made things happen. He said we had to move David to Columbia-Presbyterian Hospital (now New York-Presbyterian Hospital). I agreed and explained that it had not been possible this morning because New York was out of the paramedics' jurisdiction. I said also that David would never have survived the early morning commuter traffic across the George Washington Bridge and through the City streets. However, I told him I wanted David at Columbia as soon as it was safe to make the transfer.

Saul told me not to worry. He would take care of the arrangements. "Don't worry!" he said again. Everyone was telling me not to worry. Why was I? Saul said he would call Alice. It seems that is what we always do in medical crises. As the line in the song "White Rabbit" by Jefferson Airplane says, "Go ask Alice. I think she'll know."

Alice is Alice Prince, MD. Alice always knows what to do and whom to call to make things right. I guess she has a little magic too—maybe a lot. She had been a postdoctoral research fellow in David's laboratory in the mid-1980s. She is now a professor in Columbia's medical school and a physician at Babies and Children's Hospital there.

Alice seems to know everyone, and she carries a lot of clout. One call to Alice will set things in motion. When I became gravely ill in 1994, David called Alice. Soon I was in the emergency room being examined by an amazing physician, David Markowitz, MD. He had been a student in the medical microbiology course in which my husband lectured. My husband had also been on the PhD thesis defense committee for Dr. Markowitz's wife. I like to think that I received special attention because of this, and I guess I did in some ways, but I know in my heart that Dr. Markowitz's dedication to his profession was what really saved me.

Because David was a faculty member of Columbia University, I was entitled to a room in the McKean Pavilion—the "penthouse" of the hospital—during my illness and recovery. American heiress Sunny von Bülow was down the hall from my room. She was in a persistent vegetative state from an overdose of prescription drugs. Later President Bill Clinton was a resident while he recovered from heart surgery.

I felt special. The rooms were carpeted, the staff was attentive, and the meals were as good or better than any I have eaten in a restaurant. There was tea at three o'clock, complete with cookies and a pianist in the lounge. These were some of the perks of this special part of the hospital, and it made my having to be there more pleasant. But no amount of perks could make me better. Without the doctors and nurses and their support, I would not be writing this account. And it all started with a call to Alice.

Now another crisis, and Alice came to the rescue again. She agreed with Saul and wanted David moved to Columbia immediately. She was all business. She said she'd contact the neurologist and alert a neurosurgeon—"the best." She'd arrange medical transport and assured me that they were experts. So, while I waited for David to be out of surgery, the wheels of his transfer were in motion.

CHAPTER 6

Breathe, David, Breathe!

Hours passed, and finally Dr. Hulda pushed open the waiting room door and walked in. I was eager for this moment and dreading it just the same. Dr. Hulda was flanked by three nurses. If he had good news, he would be smiling. Right? He would have been alone. Did he think I would collapse with bad news, that I would need medical assistance? The nurses stood behind him like sentries. Bryce sat on one side of me, Sheryl on the other. I too had my defenses. *If this is a face-off, I will win*, I thought.

My mouth felt dry. I sat up straighter—composing myself, trying to control my world. I clenched my hands so tightly that my knuckles were white. Moments passed. Bryce nor Sheryl nor I said anything. Finally, I drew a breath and in a small voice asked, "How is David?"

Dr. Hulda said that David was better than before the surgery and explained the results of the operation. He said we needed to wait to see. I wrung my hands and listened intently. He said that, as he drained the hemorrhage, he found a small, nubby protrusion that he was unable to remove because blood flooding the area obscured visibility. He assured me that with time he could determine the amount of damage. I nodded and hung onto each word. I waited for him to tell me not to worry.

I wanted him to say that everything would be okay. He never did.

He said that David was on life support and that his progress was constantly being monitored.

"What does that mean?" I asked. "Life support."

He told me that David was not breathing on his own. He was attached to a respirator, a machine that breathed for him. I closed my eyes and wiped at the few tears that leaked out. I breathed deeply, willing David to do the same. My mind was crammed with so many unspoken thoughts. *This is a nightmare. I will wake up. Please let me wake up — now.*

Dr. Hulda's next words took my breath away. "David is a professor," he said. *That is not news,* I thought. He continued, "He will not want to be a vegetable." I nodded. *Of course he wouldn't. Who would?* Then Dr. Hulda said that if David did not make significant improvement by the morning—less than twenty-four hours away—he would advise removing him from life support.

David's mind exploded that morning at 7:00 a.m. Now mine did!

Remove him from life support? Vegetable? Twenty-four hours? I could not wrap my mind around those thoughts. How could Dr. Hulda even think about that? What about Terri Schiavo? She existed in a coma for nearly three years before receiving a diagnosis of a persistent vegetative state. I agreed that David wouldn't want to live, or rather not live, as a vegetable, but I could not understand why Dr. Hulda was talking about hours. Why not days? Or weeks? Why wasn't he willing to give David a chance? David was strong. Dr. Hulda recognized that when he first examined him. David was persistent. I knew he would fight with everything he had. He would not accept this state. I knew it!

I quietly nodded as thoughts whirred in my mind. *David will not be here tomorrow. He will be at Columbia-Presbyterian. I will be sure of that*, I silently promised. I was grateful that I had already called Alice.

Dr. Hulda directed me to the recovery room, where David would be for several hours. When—or if—David stabilized, he would be moved to the ICU (intensive care unit). Dr. Hulda said that I could stay in the recovery room as long as I wished. Then he left.

I made my way down the labyrinth-like hallways to the recovery room. Before entering, I put on a hospital gown, then pushed open the door. Some cubicles had the curtains pulled back, showing the people in beds; many did not. Black, white, men, women, even a child—illness is not discriminating. Everyone was sick, very sick. I scanned the room until a nurse caught my eye. He directed me to David.

I walked to David's bed, slowly, quietly, not wanting to disturb anyone. I need not have been stealthy on David's account. Nothing could rouse him. He looked gray and wounded as he lay unmoving except for the gentle rise and fall of his blanket. He was unaware of me or anything else in the room. I stared at the tube protruding from his mouth. It was attached to the machine behind his head—the one with blinking red numbers, the one making the whooshing sound, the one propelling oxygen into his lungs and allowing him to breathe. I hated that machine and I loved it. David was dependent on it to keep him alive. I ran my fingers over his hand and gently brushed his arm—careful not to disturb the tubing. I needed to touch him, to feel the warmth of him—to feel his life.

David's nurse introduced himself. His name was Gil. He was patient with me. He answered my questions, and I had many. "What is this machine for? Why is it beeping? What do these numbers mean? How can I help David? How long will he have to have the tube in his mouth? Why are those numbers changing?" My questions seemed endless, and Gil answered them all. When I did not understand, he explained again. He told me what signs to look for, and he helped me encourage David to respond to external stimuli. David needed to wiggle his toes or raise a finger on command. That would indicate brain activity.

Gil explained the numbers on the respirator, and I began to coach. "Come on, David, breathe," I whispered. I coaxed him to take deeper breaths, longer breaths. I prattled non-stop. I didn't know if he could hear me, but I never stopped imploring. "Breathe, David! Breathe! Breathe!" I told him he was strong. I told him he had to fight this battle. I repeated over and over, "Up the hill and down the hill—to Lincoln School and back!" If he heard me, he knew what I meant. It was our standing joke.

Three or four times a week, David went for runs—some long, some short. He ran through the parks of our town, all six of them. He often ran "up the hill and down the hill—to Lincoln School and back." That run was about eight miles. He'd come home drenched with sweat, exhausted but invigorated, and feeling pleased with himself. I'd scrunch up my nose and ask, "So how was your run? Where did you go?" He'd grin, and before he could answer, I'd say, "Lincoln School." David clocked over twenty miles a week. I reasoned that if he could run eight miles in one stretch and still breathe, he should surely be able to breathe while lying down in a hospital bed.

I desperately tried to reach David, who was submerged behind closed eyelids. He grasped a single thread of life. I had to strengthen that thread. I told him to fight—that I needed him. I promised I would not forgive him if he did not stay with me. I knew I was playing dirty, but the stakes were high. I had to win this match, and he had to help, and so I shamelessly threw in guilt.

I squeezed his hand over and over again in three short bursts. It was our family signal for "I love you!" Kiersten and I had invented the signal when she was a toddler. It was our secret. As we walked through the park or to the library—anywhere—I would give her hand three quick squeezes. She would squeeze back. No words passed between us, but we each knew the other had said, "I love you!" It was special having this secret. It became a family tradition. David did it, and so did our son Jared.

One day my ten-year-old granddaughter, Treska, gave my hand three short squeezes as we walked hand in hand to the swimming pool. She looked up at me with a grin on her face and asked, "Granny, do you know what that means?"

I laughed. "Your mama and I used to do that all the time."

She giggled. "I thought so."

While David lay in his bed laboriously breathing with his machines blinking and beeping, I squeezed and squeezed, and shamelessly begged him to squeeze my hand back. I was relentless. After many hours, he did—three squeezes! Maybe he squeezed because he became aware. Maybe he squeezed to make me stop pestering him. Whatever the reason, he squeezed, and my hope soared. David remembered our secret signal.

David's response encouraged me. His brain was working! He followed my directions. Gil showed me more ways to encourage David to respond. I moved my finger slowly from left to right and back again in front of David's eyes and searched for tracking movements. I commanded him to move his foot and stick out his tongue—not all at once, of course—throughout the afternoon. I continued to cheerlead, demanding these actions from David.

I slowly helped to strengthen David's thread, but he needed a rope. It would take every ounce of our combined energy to transcend the hardships and frustrations that lay ahead. David was oblivious. I too was ignorant of the difficulties we would endure. I would learn soon.

As the afternoon passed into night, David reached heightened levels of awareness. He wiggled his toes and tracked my finger with his glazed-over eyes. Then he'd close them again and retreat—to a place I could not go. The word that Dr. Hulda implanted in my head—*vegetable*—haunted me. But David was not a vegetable. He responded.

It seemed trivial to wiggle toes or track an object, but these accomplishments were monumental for David. I ran to the waiting room to tell Bryce and Sheryl of my successes. It was as though I needed them to confirm that everything would be all right. They were my witnesses. Then just as quickly I dashed back to the recovery room to continue to cheerlead. Each time David rose to the surface from whatever depth he was lurking in, I marveled and started my chant again. "Breathe! Breathe! Breathe!"

When Dr. Hulda checked on David, I excitedly showed him David's new tricks. "Look! Watch!" I begged. On command, David wiggled his toes. His eyes followed my finger—slowly, but they did. Dr. Hulda looked surprised and pleased. And now for the finale. I explained about the three short squeezes, and I urged him to watch carefully. I squeezed David's hand three times, and he squeezed my hand back, slightly . . . ever so slightly.

Dr. Hulda smiled. He had seen it! He draped his arm around my shoulder and said, "You are one lucky girl." I smiled too and waited for him to tell me that *now* everything would be okay. I was desperate for those words. But still he did not.

As Dr. Hulda left, I saw a group of hospital personnel near the door. They were staring at me and past me, at David. I recognized Janis, the emergency room receptionist, and Nina, the emergency room nurse who took such great care of David. I also saw Karen, on whose computer I first viewed David's severely damaged brain. I walked toward them. We stood hesitantly for a moment, and then we hugged. They said they heard that David had survived surgery and was still alive. They came to see for themselves.

They said no one had expected David to live, and they were excited. I could see the amazement on their faces. I was glad they came, and I was grateful they did not share their dire thoughts with me before Dr. Hulda operated on David's brain. Nina said that Dr. Faber, the emergency room doctor, wanted to come too, but the emergency room was too busy, and he sent his regards. I was amazed and impressed that these women, whom I did not know before eight o'clock this morning, showed such compassion and caring.

As the afternoon dragged on, Marie, the nurse manager of the SICU (surgical intensive care unit) said that David was ready to be moved to her care and that, as soon as he was set up and comfortable, I could join him. This was good. Right? Though we were not going home that night as I first thought when I ignorantly asked the paramedics if they could drop us home after David was seen, David was moving through the stages of healing.

When I was not in the SICU, which was rare, I fielded calls from friends and family who wanted updates on David's progress. As flights were arranged, directions to the hospital were in demand. All the loved ones trying to wend their ways from various airports around the country to the New York area had the same complaint—bad weather. The visibility at Newark

Liberty Airport was poor. Think pea soup. JFK and LaGuardia Airports in New York were no better. Both departing and arriving flights were delayed. I had barely noticed the weather, being trapped in a hospital waiting room with one dingy window.

Newark was the closest airport, but scheduling same-day flights was difficult. The exorbitant cost of fares had the travelers scrambling to find flights that would not burn holes in their pockets. Some flew into LaGuardia, and some into JFK. The lucky ones arrived in Newark.

My son Jared called to say he was flying from San Jose to JFK, the farthest airport from the hospital. Depending on traffic, it can take between one and a half and three hours to cross Manhattan into New Jersey. I didn't know how he was going to get from the airport to the hospital.

Then the phone rang again. It was Mike Marino. Soon after, Mike's wife, Angeli Kolhatcar, called. They are our racing friends. For years David and Mike raced wheel to wheel at Lime Rock Park in Connecticut, Road America in Wisconsin, Mont-Tremblant in Quebec, and Watkins Glen in upstate New York. These were just a few tracks in the Skip Barber Series, where they exhibited their driving skills.

Angeli and I cheered them—our men who loved to go fast. At the drop of the green flag, Angeli would yell, "Green! Green! Green!" into her radio, which was connected to Mike's ear. We'd watch as the cars sped from the start/finish line toward turn one—each driver determined to gain that fraction of an inch, the tenth of a second that could determine whose tires reached the checkered flag first. As Angeli shouted encouragement to Mike, I tracked David's car. With jitters, I wrung my hands, clenched my teeth, and held my breath. Until David maneuvered out of sight, I kept my eyes on his car. Then for a few seconds I'd relax, unless the radio burst into excited chatter reporting a car off-track. When David was racing and not contending for position, I enjoyed the race—clicking my stopwatch to record lap times. But when David was among the drivers fighting for the Winner's Circle, I was nervous.

I admit I was proud when David snatched a first, second, or third place. *That's my husband!* My camera snapped. It was great fun when David and Mike both did well. They often shared the podium and have the trophies to prove it.

Although I was anxious when David was on the track, I had mixed feelings. Racing was his passion, something he had dreamed of since our early years of marriage when we traipsed from racetrack to racetrack. I didn't want to dampen David's enthusiasm, yet my anxieties loomed. A serious accident would upend our lives. David had been involved in accidents, though none were his fault. Once he and Mike even crashed with a number of other cars on the straight right in front of Angeli and me. Neither that crash nor any other caused him bodily injury. On the track is where I thought our lives would come undone, not in David's home office across from our bedroom in the early morning hours. Not after tai chi exercises and chin-ups.

I was grateful when Angeli told me she was aborting her business trip in San Francisco so she could return to New York to be with David and me. When she said she was flying into JFK near the time Jared would arrive, I was relieved. One problem solved! Though Mike and Angeli had never met Jared, they said they felt they knew him. David and I had shared many Jared stories. Of course, Jared knew of our friendship with Mike and Angeli too. Strange way to finally meet.

Family and friends began to arrive at the hospital about eight o'clock that evening. The waiting room transformed into *our* reception area. My cousin Patti arrived from Florida after many weather-related flight delays. Later, she ferried out again to pick up my daughter. Kiersten suffered three flights to reach Newark Liberty. David's brothers and their wives flew into LaGuardia. Pat's brother-in-law, Scott, picked them up, as Scott's wife, Christine, drove to Newark Liberty to pick up David's father. For Christine's efforts, she was rewarded with two flat tires—compliments of New Jersey highways. Christine, ever the nurturer, brought the food—turkey and ham sandwiches with lettuce and tomato, salads, and chocolate-covered graham crackers and chocolate-covered pretzels. By the time she arrived with David's father at ten o'clock, everyone was famished. They fell upon that food.

I don't remember eating anything that day except the chocolate-covered graham crackers and pretzels. They were yummy . . . and addicting. I think the sugar sustained me as I kept vigil at David's bedside throughout the night.

CHAPTER 7

The Squeeze Game

I rarely left David's bedside. As family and friends arrived, I shared my space with them. I heard them reassure him and themselves that he would be okay. David, of course, was heedless of his well-wishers, the excitement he was causing, and the goings-on around him as he slept the slumber of ignorance. He looked terrible. His usual healthy olive complexion was gray; his eyes, sunken; his breathing, uneven and labored. Yet still we reassured him.

Most of the ICU nurses were very accommodating. They made David comfortable while attending to his many needs, and they also cared for me. They offered me water and juice and even something to eat. I declined because I didn't want them to spend their precious time on me. I appreciated their kindness, but I wanted their focus to be on David.

When evening came, one nurse wheeled in a sleeping chair for me. I was exhausted and gladly accepted, though I did not expect to sleep.

The nurses were helpful too when the rest of our family arrived, and it became congested in David's small cubicle. They stepped over us as they checked David's tubes and gauges, scrutinized his life-support machines, and monitored his level of awareness, which was near zero. They all worked with smiles on their faces and an abundance of encouraging words, except for one nurse—the Enforcer.

She was the rule sheriff. Feelings, emotions, and fears be damned! "No more than two visitors," she said. I wanted to comply, but I certainly was not leaving David's side. When my son and daughter arrived, I refused to deny them time with their father. I told the nurse about their difficult travel arrangements, how they had traveled all day, and their stressful flight delays. I promised we'd use quiet voices and that we'd be respectful of the other patients. I assured her that we'd disturb no one, and I apologized for any inconvenience my children and I might pose.

Imagine my apologizing for wanting to be with David! I told her we were staying. She refused to surrender and again directed me to the waiting room. She said that when Kiersten or Jared left, I could return. Again, I used all my persuasive skills on her and reiterated that I would not leave my husband. She wouldn't budge. As a compulsive rule-follower, I was distressed. She'd force me to disobey. I wondered if the patient were her own loved one whether she would be so eager to follow her own heartless rules. She threatened to call the nurse manager, Marie. I urged her to.

Before Marie left duty earlier that day, she wished me well. Like the other hospital personnel, Marie didn't expect David to live and bent the rules to allow us the comfort of being with him, which we desperately needed. Marie also gave me her business card and encouraged me to call her if I needed her. I would have, but it wasn't necessary. Apparently the Enforcer called because she soon left us alone, though her frown deepened. Perhaps she should consider another profession. Maybe they needed guards at Rikers Island.

I curled up on the sleeping chair. It was uncomfortable, but it allowed me to close my eyes yet monitor changes in David. Kiersten and Jared stayed by their father's bedside throughout the night, one on each side. They kept up a constant chatter, asking him if he was in pain, if he needed anything, or if he was comfortable. We used our quiet voices to whisper words of encouragement—words meant to prod him back to reality.

Of course, David never answered. He lay inert, ignorant of their ministrations, but that didn't stop them. They too believed that our words penetrated David's mind. To pass time, they caught up with each other's lives. Jared talked about his research project, his diving experiences, and his life in Santa Cruz. Kiersten told him about the many babies she had delivered, both in the clinic and on the mesa of Taos, and what her daughters were learning in school. They included David in the conversation. If he heard, he gave no indication.

As the night wore on, Kiersten and Jared devised a game to encourage their father to respond. They'd ask a question. David was supposed to squeeze their hands to answer. One squeeze meant yes. Two squeezes meant no. Surprisingly, David responded, but his answers were inconsistent. So, my creative kids reevaluated their rules. Jared went to one side of the bed, and Kiersten stayed on the other. Now when they asked a question, David was directed to squeeze Kiersten's hand for a yes answer and Jared's hand for a no answer. We were elated when David demonstrated a degree of consciousness.

They began with simple questions. Jared asked, "Dad, do I live in California?" Kiersten yelped when she received a yes squeeze. Then Kiersten asked, "Dad, do I have two sons?" Jared smiled. "I got it," he said. "Dad squeezed my hand." Not to be outdone, Kiersten quickly asked, "Dad, do I have two daughters?" A short squeeze to her hand gave her the answer she wanted. A primitive communication system was established. It was paramount, and it opened David's mind to us—if only a little.

Then it was my turn. I squeezed David's hand three times and asked if he knew what it meant. He squeezed the yes hand. Tears rolled down my cheeks. I told him what had happened. I told him that he was at Sierta Hospital, and I briefly explained the surgery. I didn't want to scare him with details and the magnitude of his crisis. I said he was recovering, and I asked if he wanted to go to Columbia-Presbyterian Hospital. No hesitation! He quickly and firmly squeezed the yes hand.

I told him not to worry—probably useless words, but it seemed the thing to say. I told him I had contacted Saul, who contacted Alice. Arrangements were being made to move him when he was stable enough to be safely transported. David seemed visibly relieved. I was grateful not to have to make this decision alone.

Though I knew it was the right thing to do, the transport scared me. I believed the worst was over. David had survived the surgery against all odds, and I thought he would recover at Sierta. I was torn by my indecision. It was a relief that David made the ultimate choice. I didn't know what was to come— neither of us did.

CHAPTER 8

Over the River

It was Friday the 14th. Everyone jokes about Friday the 13th being the unlucky day. For David and me, it was Thursday the 13th. That was the most unlucky day of our lives. Of course, if you subscribe to the "glass half full" theory, you might think it was a lucky day. After all, David survived. He beat terrible odds. He was living and breathing . . . barely. Although I knew his life was hanging by a thread, I would not believe it. Denial was my new best friend.

My eyes were red, my clothes were rumpled, and anxiety enveloped me as Friday morning dawned. The nurses attempted to wean David off the respirator. I hoped that he'd take the hint and start breathing on his own, but he didn't. As he struggled for each breath, it was obvious that life support was the tether keeping him this side of heaven—or, in this case, hell.

I remembered Dr. Hulda's term—"vegetable"—and I was again engulfed by panic. It seemed a lifetime ago that he hinted at removing David from life support if David did not breathe on his own, but it was only yesterday, less than twenty-four hours ago. I begged David to breathe. The tube remained hanging from the corner of his mouth, dragging it down—dragging me down too.

Finally, it was time for the doctors' rounds. I looked forward to Dr. Hulda's visit, hoping he would give me a positive assessment of David's condition. I hoped he'd tell me that David would soon be well. I was relieved as I watched Dr. Hulda barge through the SICU doors, his trench coat open and flowing behind him. Then I panicked. Perhaps I didn't want his news. My emotions were thread-like, stretched taut, ready to snap.

I introduced Dr. Hulda to Kiersten and Jared. I told him of the communication system they had devised—squeezing hands, which seemed to penetrate David's unconscious state. Kiersten and Jared were eager to demonstrate David's response abilities. They wanted Dr. Hulda to confirm that their father was getting better. We all hoped Dr. Hulda would say, "It's a miracle!" Though I don't believe in miracles, I wanted to be wrong.

But no miracle happened that morning. Just as an errant child ignores his mother's proud boasts, David too refused to perform. He may have been sleeping deeply after the pestering he endured through the night. Dr. Hulda saw none of David's exciting accomplishments, and I was disappointed.

Dr. Hulda needed his own proof of David's awareness. To test David's cognitive ability, he commanded him to stick out his tongue and to wiggle his fingers and toes. Attempting to get a response, Dr. Hulda flicked the bottom of David's foot. David did not react to any of these stimuli. Then Dr. Hulda said "Watch this!" as he slammed the heel of his hand, with great force, into the middle of David's chest. My jaw dropped. I'm sure David was shocked too. He nearly jumped off the bed. The punch was so mighty I thought it would break David's sternum or a rib or two. David is not an aggressive man, but I'm sure he would've returned this unwarranted gesture had he been able. I didn't understand why such force was necessary, especially since we'd told Dr. Hulda that David was responding through the night.

After the examination, I told Dr. Hulda that I planned to move David to Columbia-Presbyterian Hospital as soon as he was safely able to make the transfer. Dr. Hulda became visibly upset and urged me to reconsider. He said it was dangerous, and though I agreed, I would honor David's wishes. After all, he had squeezed the yes hand when I asked about the transfer to Columbia-Presbyterian. Though that took the burden off of me and though I was petrified of the danger to David, I would take an aggressive stance in support of the transfer.

I told Dr. Hulda that David's department chairman, Dr. Saul Silverstein, and a friend, Dr. Alice Prince, were making preparations for his transfer. Dr. Prince had arranged for a neurologist, Dr. Stephan Mayer, to accept David's case. Dr. Hulda seemed defensive. He made reference to being "out in the sticks." He was only a few miles from midtown Manhattan—certainly not the sticks. But Sierta Hospital, even with its kind and caring personnel, was not Columbia-Presbyterian, one of the best hospitals in the world.

I knew that Dr. Hulda was upset and assured him that the decision was not personal. I said that I was grateful he saved David's life, and I lightly touched his arm to calm him. As I reflect on this, I wonder—shouldn't Dr. Hulda have been comforting me? Reassuring me? Encouraging me? Didn't he understand this was the most difficult decision of my life? That I was doing my best? Instead, he firmly asserted that I was making a grave mistake. He said that David may die in transport. I knew that, but I also knew that David might die without the aggressive care provided at Columbia-Presbyterian.

Dr. Hulda continued to try to dissuade me. He said that ambulances were not the gentlest mode of transportation.

My recent firsthand experience was testimony to that fact. It is a wonder that people don't die from the ambulance ride on their way to the hospital. Maybe they do. Dr. Hulda was not appeased, even as I explained that David and I had agreed that we would always go to Columbia-Presbyterian for hospital care. I planned to keep that promise.

Finally, Dr. Hulda insisted he would only release David to a neurologist. I agreed to that. With no additional words, he left with the same flourish he had arrived, trench coat flying behind him.

I stood there, my mind spinning. What if I erred? What if David died in transport? How could I live with my decision? What if David remained at Sierta and he died without Columbia-Presbyterian's aggressive care? It was a catch-22. I called Alice. She had arranged the best transport team for David. She assured me that they make transfers every day and they were experts. Of course, I had my doubts about ambulance rides, but Alice insisted that David be moved as soon as possible. I put my faith in Alice.

I believed that David would heal quickly at Columbia-Presbyterian and return home intact. But my head was lodged in the sand, and I was in extreme denial of the seriousness of David's trauma. Some say ignorance is bliss. Well, bliss it's not, but my denial held me together in those early days.

Alice made the transfer arrangements for David. I was relieved to have her take charge. She contacted the fellow in charge of the NICU (neurological intensive care unit) at Columbia-Presbyterian. A fellow is a board-certified physician in a primary specialty, such as cardiology, who is in training for board certification in a sub-specialty, such as neurology. The fellow agreed to David's immediate transfer, and though the NICU was full, he promised to find a bed for David.

Unfortunately, it was not easy to get David released from Sierta Hospital.

Alice made several attempts to contact Dr. Hulda at Sierta to present her plan, but she was unable to reach him. Finally, when Alice used her professional title—"Dr. Prince, a professor at Columbia"—she reaped results. She explained the transfer to Dr. Hulda, but he refused to speak to the fellow in charge of the NICU. He insisted on speaking to the attending. An attending physician is also a board-certified physician and is licensed in a specialty or sub-specialty, such as pediatric cardiology. The attending acts as supervisor to fellows, residents, interns, and medical students. Attendings are ultimately responsible for the care of the patient, though most of the day-to-day and minute-to-minute decisions fall on the fellow. The attending of the NICU at Columbia-Presbyterian Hospital, Dr. Stephan Mayer, was not on call that evening, but Alice, with her wily ways, tracked him down on his cell phone. He was in a taxicab somewhere in New York City. Dr. Mayer told Alice what she already knew—that the fellows ran the NICU. However, after hearing Alice's predicament, he agreed to speak with Dr. Hulda. But since Dr. Mayer was not on call, Dr. Hulda refused to release David. Plans for transfer were reluctantly agreed upon for the following day. I was disappointed. I felt a grave urgency that David receive immediate care at Columbia.

Dr. Hulda again sought me out to attempt to dissuade me. He reminded me of how dangerous the transfer was. I listened politely, but my mind was made up. I told him that the best transport team was being sent and every precaution was being taken. I was eager for the move to be complete. Dr. Hulda seemed resigned. He was not happy that gray Friday afternoon. Again, I tried to explain but soon realized I would not see success. When Dr. Hulda departed that afternoon, I don't recall seeing him again. Frankly, I don't recall seeing any physician during the next twenty-four hours before David's transfer. How odd!

I hovered near David's bed as I waited for the transfer team. I was surprised when a nurse poked her head into David's cubicle to tell me that Dr. Haredo, Vice President of Medical Affairs at Sierta, wanted to talk with me. I thought it strange, but at the same time I was flattered. Dr. Haredo warned that David's transfer to Columbia-Presbyterian was dangerous and requested that I reconsider. I assured him that I was relying on good medical advice and though I appreciated his concern, I was adamant about the transfer. He wished me well.

Finally everything was in place, and we awaited the arrival of the transport team from Columbia-Presbyterian. The paramedics came at about 4:00 p.m. When they pushed through the doors, it was as though Superman had arrived—two Supermen, actually. One named Lou; the other, Tom.

Though they were business-like, their efficiency did not hamper their kindness. They realized I was a wreck, and their compassion for me was reassuring. They explained their work to me as they prepared David for the journey across the Hudson River. I silently prayed that I—we—had made the right decision. Their deliberate actions calmed me.

I watched as they detached David from the Sierta Hospital equipment and reattached him to the life-support machines that would sustain him until he reached Columbia-Presbyterian. I leaned against the wall to be out of their way, but I needed to be near. Their movements seemed choreographed—like a dance. It was obvious they had performed these tasks many times, and I felt that David was in the best hands. I had to trust them.

I watched David lie there—gray, barely alive, drained of every spark of energy. I felt nearly lifeless too. It was surreal, like an unending nightmare that seemed to have started a lifetime ago. However, I *was* awake and had been for about fifty-eight hours—not counting the catnaps when my eyes closed after refusing to take my command to stay alert.

The careful efforts of Tom and Lou took nearly two hours. When they finished their preparations and when the paperwork was complete, they were ready to go. David looked waxen on their gurney. They reiterated what Alice had said—that they made fragile transfers every day and that they would take good care of David. They said there was no hurry and promised to drive slowly. They would cause no undue stress to David.

They said that it would take some hours before David was settled in the NICU at Columbia-Presbyterian and that I didn't need to rush to get there. They told me to go home, freshen up, and pack clothes for the next portion of this misadventure.

It was hard to let go of David's hand. I grasped it until we reached the double doors of the SICU. Then I kissed him again and whispered that I loved him—that I always had and I always would. I said I would meet him at Columbia-Presbyterian. Then I pressed the automatic door opener for Tom and Lou and watched as they wheeled David, firmly strapped to the gurney, down the hallway. I stood there a long time and silently brushed tears from my eyes. I prayed deep in my heart that David would survive and that I really would see him again safely in New York. I didn't know how I would cope if the unthinkable happened. I knew half my life would be gone.

My entourage stared with me at the closed doors—my children, David's brothers and their wives, and David's father. My cousin Patti and her husband Bryce and our close friends Angeli and Mike joined too. We all looked lost—our arms around each other, holding each other up—watching as David was wheeled away.

I know now in retrospect that, although David's life was

initially saved at Sierta, I am not certain if it would have been again—and yet again. From my observations of the first three days of David's trauma, all of Sierta's support staff, except for the Enforcer, were attentive and caring, even personally offering their prayers for David. But the approach of the hospital, or maybe it was that of the doctor, seemed passive, reactive—not proactive. For three days, David lay in his recovery bed with only three life-support machines (respirator, blood pressure, blood/oxygen meter) supplying vital information. I never saw any machines monitoring his brain activity. Shouldn't there have been? After all, he just had brain surgery.

As far as I remember, at Sierta David never had a CT scan or an EEG after the surgery, though he spent two nights and three days there. He never left the SICU. I didn't know what to expect, and I didn't question. After all, this was my first experience with brain surgery.

Jolted with the realization that we were watching a closed door, I suggested we go to my home. I gathered my belongings from David's cubicle. Then I went in search of some very special caregivers to bid goodbye.

First I found Marie, the nurse manager. I expressed my appreciation for her compassion, understanding, and her personal interest in me when I felt lost immediately following David's surgery. I thanked her for accommodating my friends and my frenzied out-of-town family. I complimented her staff and asked her to tell them. I also told her of the Enforcer, the nurse who caused such distress. I hadn't planned to mention her because I didn't want to leave on a negative note, but I felt Marie should be alerted to the nurse's attitude. I felt that the Enforcer's behavior was unwarranted and shouldn't be inflicted on any family embroiled in the unhappy business of keeping a life-watch of a loved one. Marie knew immediately of whom I spoke, and she promised to speak with her. It seems the Enforcer had wreaked havoc on hapless families before mine.

After hugging Marie goodbye, I walked the long, maze-like hallways to the recovery room to bid farewell to Gil, David's first post-surgery nurse. I thanked Gil for his special care. He was my first teacher in this process. And he recognized my desperate need to be at David's bedside. I wanted Gil to know that I would always remember his kindness.

I had two more visits to make before I left the hospital. I went in search of Nina and Janis. How lucky I was that they were the first persons I met at Sierta Hospital. Nina was where I left her—in the emergency room. She told me I was strong and how she admired me. I didn't *feel* strong. I was falling apart—barely holding myself together—but she made me feel good. She said again how lucky David and I were. I smiled and hugged her.

Janis was not at her desk. While it was Nina who cared for David, it was Janis who cared for me. It was Janis who gave me her seat behind the reception area and allowed me to use her phone. It was Janis who distracted me from the dire situation playing out in the emergency room across the hall. It was Janis who sat with me during her fifteen-minute break on Friday afternoon, assured me that everything would be okay, and told me that her prayer group was praying for David's recovery. When I did not find her, I was disappointed, but I wrote my words of gratitude and left them on her desk.

My errands done, it was time to leave Sierta. We piled into cars for the drive home. I began this journey in an ambulance early Thursday morning. I was leaving the hospital more than sixty hours later as darkness fell, but I was only at the beginning of this nightmare.

CHAPTER 9

What a Mess!

As we drove home through the darkness, it felt strange not having David with me to show off our new home to our family. Although we'd lived in our home for five years, no one had yet visited. Now everyone was here, but the fun had been stripped away. David was missing from the welcoming committee.

It may seem odd that none of our family had visited in five years, but there were good reasons. It was difficult for David's father to make the ten-hour car trip from Erie. Kiersten and David's brothers all had families, while we were empty nesters. So, we traveled to them. During holiday breaks, we sometimes flew to New Mexico to visit Kiersten and her family. It was cost-efficient for them. And since Jared often flew from Santa Cruz to join us at Kiersten's in Taos, it was unnecessary for him to journey across the continent to New Jersey. Often, we'd meet David's brothers' families at his father's house in Erie. They were juggling their children's school and sports schedules and found it difficult to make the trek to New Jersey.

The house was a mess—sort of a controlled disarray, but still a mess. We had hired a company to paint the interior of our house just after Christmas, and it hadn't been restored yet. David and I had decided to get the house painted when a trip to Puerto Peñasco, Mexico, with my brother John and his wife, Carol, fell through.

At least once a year, John and Carol would pull up to the north exit of the Sky Harbor Airport in Phoenix. David would squeeze our luggage into their trunk—around coolers, bags of food, beach chairs, towels, flippers, and snorkels. Then we would squeeze ourselves into the car for the four-hour-plus trip into Mexico.

I loved the drive through Organ Pipe Cactus National Monument. The organ pipe cactus is rare in the United States except in southern Arizona. My favorite cacti are the saguaro and the cholla. They are especially beautiful when they are in full bloom. The cacti, together with the low-slung mountains and the puffy, white clouds surrounding them, are magical. Usually the trip exceeded four hours because of my shouts of "Stop!" from the back seat. My brother was patient with me as I ventured into the desert with my camera—capturing the indescribable beauty and savoring the quiet.

It was fun to drive through Ajo too, which means "garlic" in Spanish. Despite its name, I've never smelled garlic in this town forty-three miles from Mexico. When we crossed the Mexican border, my pulse quickened. We entered another world—an older world.

I loved Mexico. I loved our little bungalow on the water's edge and the vendors, who came right up to our door with their trays of silver necklaces, bracelets, and other trinkets. "For you—almost free!" they'd say with an entreating smile. I loved the thrill of parasailing, which Carol cajoled us into trying on one trip. She has not yet convinced us to try the banana boat. The rubber raft-boat shaped like a yellow banana crashing on the waves looked painful. I loved happy hour on the Playa Bonito overlooking the Sea of Cortés with its stunning sunsets as we all gorged on shrimp and quesadillas. David rarely drinks anything but wine, but in PP, as we fondly call it, he would indulge in margaritas, which he swore were the best.

Our visits to Puerto Peñasco were pure fun, and I loved the escape from the hustle-bustle of the New York City area. Most of all, I loved spending carefree time with David, John, and Carol—my PP pals.

Unfortunately, at the end of 2004 I was unable to find an affordable flight to Phoenix, so we all reluctantly postponed our Christmas escape to Puerto Peñasco until April 2005. Instead, David and I used the time to have the walls of our house painted.

It was fortunate our plan to visit Puerto Peñasco over the holidays was thwarted. On December 27th, our phone rang. My brother John, with a cracked voice, told me his bad news. His twenty-four-year-old son, Little John, had had a "brain bleed." My brother told me the doctors said Little John had a 50 percent chance to live. They said he had suffered a traumatic brain injury (TBI). I had never heard of that before, and my brother explained that something burst in Little John's head. The intense pressure was causing unknown damage and was potentially life-threatening.

Little John lived. But he was left with major obstacles to overcome. His brain injury, the cause of which the doctors were never able to explain, left him with balance and speech impairments. He battles these still. But my happy-go-lucky, devil-in-his-eyes nephew will not give up. He often remarks, "This is a small speed bump in the road of life." Some speed bump! Some optimism! Some kid!

I hate to imagine what would've happened if we had been in Mexico—out of phone contact and four hours away. But we weren't, and John and Carol rushed their son to the hospital in time—time that was crucial to the amount of damage sustained.

Since we did not go to Puerto Peñasco, David and I spent Christmas at home. On Christmas Eve, we had a picnic on the floor in front of our fireplace. On a blue-checkered tablecloth, I set bowls of jumbo shrimp and cocktail sauce, grilled sausage slices with horseradish and mustard dipping sauces, cubes of cheese with crackers and bread wedges, a glass of red wine for David, and a non-alcoholic beer for me. No margaritas or quesadillas; no sun, sand, and sea; no cholla or red mountains; and no brother to tease or a sister-in-law to have girly-girl talks with. Yet our picnic was a cozy affair—calm and relaxing with no pressure. David and I spent the evening talking in the dimly lit room with the flames of the fireplace dancing in the background. We talked about everything. We even talked each other into hiring a painter to paint the interior of the whole house over our holiday break. Fat chance to schedule a painter over the holidays, we thought, but we were lucky.

On Christmas morning, David and I woke late. We leisurely opened our presents. David gave me scented things—perfumes, candles, and oils—and a beautiful silver necklace. For David's long runs to Lincoln School and back, I gave him winter running clothes—pants and jacket, hooded sweatshirts, and special underwear. Snow and cold did not hinder David's passion for running, and I wanted him to be warm.

I encouraged David to try on his new running clothes. He did, then goofily ran up and down our short hallway, demonstrating his running form until I caught the perfect pose on my camera. He was a good sport and accommodated my silly request. I am glad he did. Those were the last pictures I have of him from when life was normal.

I hung those pictures on the walls in each of David's hospital rooms. I wanted everyone—doctors, nurses, technicians, therapists, and other patients—to see who the "real" David was. I also thought it was important for our family and friends to hold onto the memory of the vibrant David we all knew. I didn't want them to think of him as the helpless patient he had become. That was *not* David! His present condition was a "bump in the road"—temporary. (I often wonder how to quantify temporary. Dictionary.com states that temporary is "not permanent." Unfortunately, the dictionary does not state *how long* temporary is. So far, our temporary has been more than twelve years. That's a long temporary!)

David's brother, Tom, encouraged us to fly to Detroit for New Year's. We weighed the options—reassemble the house or fly on a last-minute whim to spend the holiday with David's brothers and their families. David's father was there too. The balance fell heavily on flying to Detroit, and so we did.

We enjoyed a quiet New Year's Eve. We went to dinner with the family. We returned to Tom's house and laughed and talked around the fireplace, and we danced to '60s music. We slept late the next morning, had a quick brunch, and caught an early afternoon flight home. I am thankful for that spur-of-the-moment trip. It was the last time that David's family saw him BT (before trauma). Life would be very different in New Year 2005, and it would not include dancing.

The year 2004 had been peppered with stress, and David and I had been happy to bid it farewell. David's phrase for the new year was "2005 is going to be a great year!" and we looked forward to it. But if we thought that 2004 was stressful, we would soon learn a new meaning for the word *stress*.

As I opened the door of my home to my family for this unexpected visit, it was with mixed feelings—happy with our color choices, embarrassed that the house was not perfect with everything in its proper place, and sad, so sad, that David was not with me to share the fun of welcoming our family to our home, even in its temporarily messy state.

It seems silly now that I worried about the disarray in my house. I apologized for the mess—the piles of books on the floor waiting to be alphabetized, the framed photos and scented candles all needing to be re-shelved. Of course, everyone brushed aside my apologies. I promised I would put everything in order, and I did too, but not until three months passed. It was more a promise, I think, to myself.

CHAPTER 10

Packing for Uncertainty

I welcomed everyone into my newly painted home and made more apologies for the mess left by the painters. We weren't staying long—just time enough for me to take a much-needed shower. As I climbed the stairs to the third floor, a melancholy I didn't anticipate crept over me. I desperately tried to remain in control, but suppressed emotions bobbed to the surface. As I stepped into our bedroom, the images of David's pain as he writhed on the bed clutching his head assaulted me. It was as though I were replaying a very bad movie, every single scene of it in slow motion. I was grateful to be away from the watchful eyes of my family and friends. I slammed the bathroom door shut, turned on the water, and stepped into the shower—my great escape. My tears mingled with the warm water and splashed down the drain. That was my first release—the first tears I allowed myself. I wish that the consequences of David's TBI could be as easily washed away.

When my emotions drained and I regained my composure, I put on lipstick, eye shadow, and liner to help conceal my breakdown. I threw clothes into my backpack—jeans, shirts, socks, and underwear. I tucked in my hairdryer and flat iron, my toothbrush, and a couple pair of pajamas. Then I trudged downstairs.

Everyone had gathered around the fireplace. Some were perched on my blue leather couches. They rehashed the events of the past two and a half days and wondered what the next days would bring. Before we left for the hospital, I sorted through the food in the refrigerator, packing what was salvageable into a cooler to take with me. The rest I tossed into the trash. Then I packed up my computer and the books I was currently reviewing for my column Teacher's Pets. I also packed my registration materials for Kindling Words: The Retreat, a retreat/conference for writers, illustrators, editors, and agents, which was to be held at Lake George, New York, in two weeks.

I took the position of registrar for Kindling Words in 1998, and since September, I had been preparing for the annual end-of-January conference. I felt a responsibility to my co-organizers and the retreat registrants to process last-minute registrations, despite this emergency in my life. The retreat director said not to worry, but I worried anyhow. I did not want to let anyone down. I was the only one with the database containing all of the information. I felt compelled to iron out all last-minute details. I had to alert the director of any food restrictions, finish room assignments, and compile the sweatshirt orders. I also had to complete the bio/intro book, which was a feature that I launched in 1998. After I returned from the hospital, I completed what needed to be done each night between 12:00 and 1:00 a.m. so that the conference could go on without a glitch . . . without me. It made me feel better; it made me feel worse.

With everything packed, we piled into cars and headed toward New York City. Tom drove my car. As we neared the City, the drivers stayed connected by cell phones. No one but me knew how to get there. We did not want to get lost.

Driving into New York City on a Saturday night is challenging. We crossed the George Washington Bridge and wended our way down Broadway, edging our cars through the narrow streets without incident and finally parking them in David's underground parking garage, only two blocks from his lab and office. When Tom pulled the keys from the ignition, I breathed a sigh of relief. I did not see my car again for weeks.

Two of David's graduate students, Brenda Perez and Azeem Siddique, and two of his postdoctoral research fellows, Valerie Weaver Grosso and Mladin Tomich, met us outside the garage on Hudson Terrace. Amidst their many questions, their curiosity, and their deep concern to understand what had happened to their mentor, they guided me to my new home and helped me move in.

Saul, my magic man, was responsible for my accommodations while David was a "guest" of the hospital. Kiersten, Jared, and I moved into a very comfortable apartment in the student dorms only blocks from the hospital. We unpacked the food and stored it on the pantry shelves. We found a well-stocked refrigerator. Valerie had shopped that morning and stuffed the refrigerator with fresh vegetables and fruits, bread and cheeses, and orange juice. What a welcome surprise!

This was not a typical dorm room. It was actually a suite overlooking the Hudson River set aside for visiting professors and dignitaries. The view of the George Washington Bridge and the Palisades of New Jersey was captivating, especially at night, as snowflakes the size of nickels fell in a January blizzard. The bridge lights hung like diamonds shimmering in the night sky. It was magical, and we needed magic. In the early morning hours, I'd press my forehead against the window, lost in thought, my eyes gazing at the cars below as they inched their way through the maze of roads leading to the Henry Hudson Parkway or Riverside Drive. They looked like ants, scurrying, going nowhere. I too was going nowhere—not for a long time.

Although David and I live only twenty-five miles from the hospital, the commute can be time-consuming. A normally thirty-minute drive can easily take twice that long or longer, depending on traffic. Not having to commute was a gift. The commute would have deterred me from going home. Sleeping on the waiting room couches, though not appealing, would have become my way of life for the next weeks.

Kiersten and Jared lived with me for the next five weeks, but unfortunately Tom and Kathy, Pat and Patrice, and Hank each had tickets back to a normal reality. Their flights were on Monday and Tuesday. I dreaded their departures. I felt my world narrowing, and I was overwhelmed with pain and uncertainty, but there were still seeds of hope.

CHAPTER 11

Hearths

After I settled into the apartment, I began to panic. Although it had only been two hours since I last saw David, it seemed eons ago. With an urgency I could not quell, I threw on my coat. Everyone else put on theirs too, and we hurried the few blocks to the hospital.

I pushed through the revolving door at the Milstein Building of Columbia-Presbyterian Hospital and got directions from a guard named Paris. With passes in hand, we squeezed into an elevator. I pressed the button for the fourth floor. This world—so alien to me then—would become my second home over the next few weeks.

When I stepped off the elevator, I searched for the NICU. The double doors were foreboding, and I pushed them open with trepidation. I walked to the nurse's station, almost on tiptoe, not wanting to disturb the patients. I glanced into each room hoping to catch a glimpse of David. A nurse looked up from her station, smiled, and directed me to a cubicle. Without my asking, she knew. I was the new kid on the block because David was.

David's curtain was drawn, and the nurse said that he was still being assessed. I carefully pushed the curtain aside. David was attached to a multitude of machines—unlike at Sierta.

After only minutes, the nurse walked me to the waiting room. She promised to alert me when David could have visitors.

The waiting room was huge. There were couches in clusters —some small, some large, each with a table in the middle. The groupings reminded me of *The Clan of the Cave Bear* by Jean Auel that I read many years ago. Auel wrote about prehistoric man, the Clan people. She told how each family gathered around its hearth at night. The hearth was a private place. It was considered impolite to peer into someone else's hearth. That's the way it felt in the waiting room too. Family and friends gathered in a couch section, their hearth, with little awareness of the others. Each group was engrossed in its own troubles. It did seem rude to steal glances into someone else's hearth, to invade another group's pain and misery. The waiting room had an abundance of tears and anguish. I'm sure it also saw happiness and joy, and that thought was refreshing. At least there was hope for some of us.

I waited while the doctors poked and probed and tested and did whatever they do when a new patient becomes theirs. Periodically, when my patience wore thin and I wondered if the nurses, with all their duties, had forgotten me, I'd peek through the double doors. David's curtain remained drawn.

The waiting room emptied as the night wore on. Weary visitors went home, expecting to return the next day to continue their vigils. I needed to escape too and curled up on a couch away from my family. They sat in a couch cluster consoling each other, but I needed space—to be quiet, to think. I turned inward, wrapping myself in a cocoon, hoping to blot out this surreal scene. Tears again slipped down my face. As I wept, I silently begged to know why this was happening. David didn't deserve this. We didn't. I remained in a fetal position until the nurse came to take me to David.

Time to brush away the tears and put a smile on my face. Time to pretend that everything would be all right. I took a deep breath, pushed through the double doors, and walked down the hallway. Kiersten and Jared followed. David's brothers and father waited in the waiting room. They respected our privacy and they would join us soon.

All of the patient rooms were on the left, and David's was halfway down the corridor. The nurses' station was directly across from David's cubicle, and that comforted me. I stood at the entrance of David's space. That's all it was—space only for a bed, a chair, and many machines. I stared and drew in a breath.

Machines buzzed. The respirator, also called the breathing machine, hissed—a welcome sound. Its rhythmic hiss was testimony that David was alive. But it also meant that he was unable to breathe on his own—an unwelcome thought. The tube from the breathing machine securely placed in David's mouth forced oxygen into his lungs and removed carbon dioxide. Ideally the machine is used only a short time—until the patient is able to breathe on his or her own. That the respirator was keeping David alive was a scary reality. I wondered, what if his brain did not remember how to breathe . . . what then? What if he did not get enough oxygen? Is that what Dr. Hulda meant when he suggested David might become a vegetable?

My eyes were drawn to a machine behind David's bed. It was a bedside monitor. Red numbers flashed on its screen. Green streaks zipped across in a zig-zag pattern. Blue, yellow, and white lines raced to the edge of the screen and then began again. They seemed endless. I didn't know what the lines or numbers meant, but after days of constant questioning, I learned. David was attached to the monitor by wires called leads. They are sensitive to even the slightest change in a bodily function. The monitor kept track of his heart and breathing rates, his blood pressure, body temperature, and even the amount of oxygen in his blood. I knew the safe ranges at which I could relax, and I knew the danger levels. When a lead sensed a dangerous change in David's body, it sent a signal to the monitor. Another monitor kept in the nurse's station beeped an alarm, which usually sent the nurses scurrying to David's cubicle.

David also had an intravenous infusion pump (IV) inserted into a vein in his hand. It regulated the amount of liquids, usually medicines, infused directly into his vein. He had a variety of other monitors attached to him too. Though I never learned what they all were, I was mesmerized by them. David's room at Sierta was stark in comparison. As my eyes adjusted to the assault of machinery, I watched David from the foot of the bed—his chest rising and falling in a rhythm set by his respirator. He looked peaceful. I entered silently.

I need not have worried about being quiet. David wasn't disturbed by me. His coma-induced sleep protected him from much of the world. I wanted to shake him awake. I wanted to scream, "David, talk to me! Hear me! See me! I need you!" But he slept on. I kissed his gray cheek and rubbed his cold arm. I held his hand and repeated, "David, you will get better. David, I love you. Please fight! Can you hear me?" I prattled non-stop about anything—nonsense probably, but I knew I had to keep up the banter. I knew he'd hear me, somewhere deep in his consciousness.

The National Institute of Neurological Disorders and Stroke defines coma as "a profound or deep state of unconsciousness. An individual in a state of coma is alive but unable to move or respond to his or her environment." It does not, however, state that a patient is unaware.

When David's mother, Lydia, was dying of cancer in 1979, she fell into a coma. We all gathered in Erie to be with her.

As Lydia slept, her doctor insisted that she was unaware and unable to comprehend. With careless abandon, he discussed in her presence her prognosis and his inability to cure her. The doctor's action troubled us. David and I believed his mother was aware at some level, and on the night before she died, she proved it. I gently squeezed Lydia's hand, and I asked her to squeeze mine back. She did. I became greedy and asked for three squeezes. She rewarded me again. Through the night we made a game of it, requesting a random number of squeezes, and she complied. Sometimes she would drift away, as though it were hard work, and I guess it was. Spending those hours with my mother-in-law convinced me that patients in a coma experience awareness.

Another incident happened the next morning when Lydia's breath became shallow, and it was obvious she was hanging onto life by a mere thread. I'm sure she heard her husband assure her that he would be okay and that it was all right for her to go. At the moment he kissed her goodbye, a bright ray of light streamed through the window on that sunless morning of December 27th. It shone directly on Hank and Lydia as he kissed her. It warmed the room and everyone in it. Then Lydia took her last breath as the light and the warmth ebbed away with her life. If I had not been at her bedside with nine other family members as witnesses, I doubt that I would have believed it, but I was witness, and I do believe that she heard Hank.

While David was in a coma, I believed without a doubt that he was aware of his surroundings, at least at a minimal level. So I talked to him, and I encouraged him in an attempt to reach him.

CHAPTER 12

Rip Van Winkle

Being able to walk to the hospital from our apartment in Bard Hall in five minutes allowed me to stay with David the entire day. From seven o'clock in the morning until eleven or twelve o'clock at night, I stayed by his side. The hours blended into days. The days passed in a blur. Except for my hour-and-a-half break during the nurses' evening shift change, there was no life for me outside the hospital.

Each morning, I awoke in darkness. It took only a moment to realize where I was and why. Reality struck hard! I crept from the unfamiliar bed and tiptoed to the bathroom. It was an unspoken agreement that I would use the shower first. Unlike my home with its four bathrooms, too many for David and me but a welcome asset when we entertained overnight company, there was only one bathroom in the apartment. Everyone respected my need to be ready first—to get to the hospital early. I would have been unable to contain myself if I had to wait.

Kiersten and Jared did not mind sleeping a few extra minutes as I showered, dressed, and dashed out the door, down the elevator, past the guard who barely acknowledged me, and walked the few blocks to the hospital. I was anxious until I reached David's cubicle. Though I didn't really relax, I felt more at ease and more in control when I was with David. It was a false sense of security—a delusion. I had no more control of David's well-being than I did of the sun rising or stars appearing at night, but it was a welcome delusion.

Around seven o'clock each morning, as the night nurses completed their chores and the day shift nurses arrived, I entered the NICU. The nurses welcomed me. They apprised me of David's condition. They were cheery no matter how tired they were.

Though it was morning, David slept on. There were no visible windows in the room, making it difficult to discern night from day even for those of us who were not struggling with consciousness. With no sense of night or day, David's circadian rhythm was interrupted. The constant buzzing of machines, the ceaseless noise of the public address system paging doctors or announcing meetings, and the hum of the nurses' voices as they attended to their patients were not conducive to sleep, yet David slept.

Sleeping or not, David could not escape my chatter. "Good morning!" I said. "How are you? I missed you." I massaged his arms and squeezed his hands. "Did you sleep well?" I asked. "Hmm, guess so! You're still sleeping," I answered myself. Then I checked the machines. "Come on, sleepyhead. Wake up!" I coaxed. "I want to talk with you." I examined his face for any discernible differences and checked all the lines feeding into him. "Don't you think you've slept enough? You'll turn into Rip Van Winkle, and we both know you don't look good with a beard." You would think he would have awakened long enough to cease my incessant chatter, to send me away, to ask how anyone could sleep with my babbling. But he didn't. He slept on, and I continued my chatter—coaxing him to get better—begging him to wake up, pleading with him to look at me, smile at me, talk to me. But he slept on.

The doctors examined David—hordes of them. Columbia-Presbyterian Hospital is a teaching hospital. I remembered from the time I had been "incarcerated" there many years ago when my knee reflexes were all the buzz on McKean Pavilion. Swarms of students came then to test their reflex hammers on the deep tendons of my knees. They tapped their tomahawk-looking instruments on my knee, and my foot would fly off the bed toward the ceiling—well, at least three inches. It was comical. It was also embarrassing because I hadn't shaved my legs before going to the emergency room. Who would've thought that my knees would become a center attraction?

When the doctors and students descended on David's room, I squeezed into the corner. They checked his ability to respond. They discussed his progress and lack of it. They gave the same commands to David each time: "Raise two fingers." "Stick out your tongue." "Flex your toes."

As the weeks passed and the doctors and students grew accustomed to me, they solicited my observations. Since I spent every moment with David, I was able to add valuable information about his progress—insight they couldn't possibly glean in a ten-minute exam. I knew what they were looking for, so I rehearsed David. Our preparations reminded me of a child studying for the weekly spelling test—spelling and writing words countless times to commit them to memory. David repeatedly practiced my commands, and when he demonstrated his skills for his audience, I was proud—as proud as any teacher whose student performed well in an evaluation. And when he did not, well, I was disappointed and I was worried.

Each day brought more technicians, more tests, and more needles. I wasn't alarmed because hospitals are known for endless testing. I prayed the tests would prove that David was getting better.

Technicians poked one of David's fingers every few hours with a lancet. They tested his blood for hyperglycemia (too much sugar) and hypoglycemia (too little sugar). Either of these conditions could pose complications. Though David's blood sugar level was always within the safe range, the technicians kept a steady vigilance. Fortunately, they varied their poking, but despite their consideration, David's fingers looked like pincushions.

Whenever a nurse or doctor suspected seizure activity in David's brain, an EEG (electroencephalogram) was ordered. An EEG is a test that detects abnormalities in the brain. One day an electroneurodiagnostic technician attached about thirty small, flat metal discs (electrodes) to David's scalp with a sticky gel. It took the technician nearly thirty minutes to secure the electrodes. My incessant questioning didn't help his speed, but he was patient with me and answered my questions.

When the electrodes were in place, he wrapped David's head. The turban-like covering made David look strange. The technician said the covering was to secure the electrodes and protect the wires so David couldn't pull them out, but David tried and succeeded a number of times anyway. The wires attached to the electrodes edged out from the covering and led to the recording machine behind his bed. The electrodes detected the electrical impulses in David's brain and recorded his brainwave patterns. A camera was directed at David, allowing his movements to be monitored from a room in the bowels of the hospital. David endured several EEGs during his stay in the NICU.

CHAPTER 13

Campuses

When I think of university campuses, I think of grassy hillocks with low buildings. I think of students purposefully strolling under trees and heading to classes. I think of the University of California at San Diego (UCSD) near the Pacific Ocean, with palm trees swaying and sweet-smelling eucalyptus trees making small groves of welcome shaded areas. David did his postdoctoral work there for four glorious years—not long enough for me. I could have lived a lifetime there. I think of the University of Rochester, where David did his graduate work in microbiology and earned his PhD degree. I remember the ground-level windows of our garden apartment in Whipple Park, a graduate and medical student housing complex not far from campus. I think of the University of Pittsburgh too, but with none of the images of the grassy campuses. Pitt is located in urban Pittsburgh. David earned his BS degree there, and I remember Pitt with happy thoughts of fraternity parties at the Phi Kappa Theta house and football games at Pitt Stadium.

I have fond memories of parties and dinners at fellow graduate students' apartments or at the homes of postdocs (postdoctoral research scientists) or professors at the University of Rochester. On the campuses, everything and everyone was nearby. We lived only miles from each other, making it easy to get together.

I remember our good friends, Jeannie and Tom, who lived across the street from us in Whipple Park. The long cold winters there made us all stir-crazy by the time we saw the first daffodil of spring. One Saturday night, David and I hosted a party, and Jeannie and Tom were there, of course. As the night wore on, Jeannie decided to check on her children and their babysitter. Instead of using the conventional means of departure—the door—Jeannie hefted herself through the garden apartment window, spilling not a drop of her precious Carlo Rossi chianti. (On graduate student salaries, we were frugal and not very discriminating.) I still laugh when I remember this scene. Click! No doubt a Kodak memory from the 1970s.

David and I hosted our share of parties in San Diego too. Our small, buttercup-yellow house, which we rented for a year, had a real wood-burning fireplace and overlooked the ocean. I loved it, even with its holey roof. In some rooms, I could see white clouds floating overhead in the blue sky. I was grateful that it did not often rain in Southern California, but when it did, I simply put out pails—about five of them.

Though the winters in San Diego were mild, that didn't stop me from lighting the fireplace every chance I got—and especially when we had a party. We didn't need it for warmth, but it lent a welcoming ambiance and harbored many stories. One favorite is a tale about Jared's hamster, Tick-Tock, who escaped his habitat and became trapped behind the walls of the fireplace. Fortunately, the fireplace was unlit, and we soon rescued him. His rapidly beating heart and twitching whiskers were his only signs of distress. Oh, there were good parties around that fireplace, but most of our parties were at the beach circling a fire ring, with lots of good talk, yummy food, special friends, and many bottles of Carlo Rossi.

Columbia University Medical Center (CUMC), where David's lab was located, is on the north end of Manhattan at 168th Street and Fort Washington Avenue. It is only a block from Broadway and ten blocks south of the George Washington Bridge. David's building, the Armand Hammer Health Sciences Center, is in a neighborhood community where Spanish dominates English. The Hammer building is surrounded by apartment houses, stores, schools, subway lines, and churches. Grass and trees are mostly confined to the parks dotting the community.

CUMC has an intense and exciting atmosphere, but its locale is not like the college campuses of my memory. Because of CUMC's urban location and our children, it was difficult for us to find appropriate housing near the university. Many professors opted to raise their children in the suburbs, with their grassy yards. We too elected to live in the suburbs. By choosing suburbia, we forfeited the out-of-the-lab camaraderie—the parties—that were more prevalent on our other campuses. The living radius was ten to as far as forty miles from CUMC. Professors were spread throughout the metropolitan New York area, including New Jersey. That made it difficult to socialize often.

Of course, there were dinner parties at the Faculty Club or at a New York City restaurant, like Isabella's on the Upper West Side, to entertain a speaker, to celebrate the successful defense of a graduate student's thesis, to acknowledge the retirement of a faculty member, or to host a formal affair honoring a colleague or fellow scientist. My favorite event was the black-tie dinner-dance at St. Patrick's Cathedral. How elegant! I felt like a princess as the valet whisked away my little white Miata convertible, and David and I ascended the stone steps and passed through the cathedral's great doors. It felt like I was in a castle. The event was a Columbia fundraiser, and they raised plenty, since each plate was worth one thousand dollars! We were the grateful guests of a professor friend and his spouse. It was a magical evening.

Though I knew David's colleagues, had had dinner with them and their spouses and had seen them in the hallways or elevators of the Hammer Health Sciences Center, we did not "party." I did not know them well. David's hospitalization would soon change that.

On Sunday, January 16th, the people in David's lab asked if they could visit him. I declined their requests. I didn't believe they realized the severity of David's trauma. How could they? I knew David wouldn't want his lab to see him in this unprofessional and compromised state, so I barred all visitors, except for the closest of family and friends. Though I realized that his lab wanted to show their respect and be reassured that their mentor was still able to advise them, it would take two months before those visits happened. When I finally allowed visits, David was still a scary site.

David's colleagues did not request permission to visit—they came. Grown men stood at David's bedside, holding back tears or letting them unashamedly roll down their cheeks as they told me how much they loved David. Yes, many of them used the word "love," which of course unleashed my own tears. I was amazed and moved by the sincerity of these men, whom I knew as well-clad scientists in suits and ties over polite dinner talk. I have the greatest respect for David as a husband, as a scientist, and as a person. I admire his very capable, intelligent mind, but I did not realize to what extent his colleagues did too. I was not embarrassed by my tears, which flowed freely as I listened to his colleagues' testimonials about him, and I was proud.

Some scientists came with whispering voices, saying how important David was to them and that they missed him. Saul, David's department chairman and good friend, came daily with his no-nonsense voice, his jocular manner, and his demands that David return to the laboratory—he was needed there.

In the early '80s, when David was fairly new to Columbia University, Saul and David would slip out of their labs and cross the street to the basement gym at Bard Hall to play handball. Though Saul tried his best to beat David, David usually won. They played once or twice a week. When Saul first visited David in the NICU, he glanced at him, nodded his head slowly, and quipped, "I can probably beat him now." Only Saul would be so irreverent. I laughed, and David would have too if he could've heard.

Dr. Dan Fine came too, with his wife, Joan. Dan called nearly five times a day, hoping for a turn of events, some good news, a miracle. Though his calls tapered off as the weeks dragged on, I knew Dan was only a speed-dial call away, and that comforted me. His respect and love for David made me proud.

Dan was a National Institutes of Health (NIH) Senior Fellow in David's lab in the late '80s. He wanted to expand his knowledge in the field of molecular genetics. It was inevitable that David and Dan would become part of each other's life. One summer, we attended a party at Dan's country home. Dan spoke of graduate school at the University of Pittsburgh. During that same time, David was an undergraduate at Pitt, and I worked in the Registrar's Office. It was probable that David and Dan had passed each other many times.

Shortly after Dan completed his work in David's laboratory, he moved to UMDNJ (University of Medicine and Dentistry of New Jersey, now Rutgers School of Medicine). Dan was recruited as professor and chairman of the Department of Oral Biology and director of the Center for Oral Infectious Diseases.

David and Dan not only became close friends, but they also became collaborators. Together they studied a bacterium that causes periodontal disease. Some of David's postdocs and students graduating with their PhDs from his laboratory crossed the Hudson River to join Dan's lab or department. Paul Goncharoff was such a postdoc. Former graduate students Helen Schreiner and Scott Kachlany joined the faculty of Dan's department.

Of course, not all of David's lab members migrated to UMDNJ. David has overseen the work of over ninety PhD students, postdoctoral fellows, undergraduates, and high school students. Each came out a little older and a lot wiser. Jim Wilson is an associate professor at Villanova University. David Bechhofer is a professor at Mount Sinai School of Medicine in New York City. Elaine Sia is a professor at the University of Rochester, spending her days walking the same campus that David did when he was working on his PhD degree. Oliver Jovanovic is an instructor at Columbia University. Paul Planet is an assistant professor at the Perelman School of Medicine at the University of Pennsylvania and sees patients at the Children's Hospital of Philadelphia. Valeri Thomson was the director of the Immediate Science Research Opportunity Program at Bard College, the same college from which my daughter and my granddaughter graduated. Valeri is currently principal of the Bard High School Early College Queens in New York City.

While David slept, many visitors stopped by, filling the fourth floor NICU waiting lounge. I was grateful for their company and the support they offered. Of course, my daughter and son were there. They put their lives on hold for nearly five weeks to encourage their father's healing. My cousin Patti and her husband, Bryce, kept vigil with us too. So did my cousin, Kathy, her husband, Sam, and their daughter, Kayla, who were frequent visitors. When David's family returned home the Monday after the first surgery, I was relieved to have my cousins prop me up. We commandeered a large section of the waiting room and made it ours as we settled there each day. Oh the party we could have had under happy circumstances! I relied on the support of my community—family and friends— again and again.

CHAPTER 14

Surprises

When David left Sierta Hospital, I believed he was on the road to recovery. I thought he would calmly and steadily climb out of the abyss he had unexpectedly fallen into, but I never realized how long his recovery would take, or how much he would endure—how much we each would endure—as he slowly and uncertainly made his way to consciousness. I thought, *Okay, he survived brain surgery. Remarkable! Now he will rest and get better.* That's how I thought it should be. One brain surgery should last a lifetime. If you should ever have the sad fortune to need one, one is definitely enough!

I am not an ignorant person, though I have been known to emulate an ostrich on occasion. Perhaps my head was buried in the sand because I have no recollection of any doctor at Sierta discussing additional procedures—definitely not another brain surgery. Not even a hint.

I knew David remained in danger. It was obvious. Dr. Hulda made it clear when he suggested that David might succumb to a vegetative state, but I don't recall his ever implying a need for more surgery. In fact, David never even had a CT scan, a PET (positron emission tomography) scan, an MRI (magnetic resonance imaging), or an EEG while at Sierta Hospital for the three days following his surgery. Naturally, I believed the worst had passed. The blood from David's brain hemorrhage had been evacuated, and the pressure was easing. I understood his recovery would take time, but I was shocked when I learned at Columbia-Presbyterian that David was facing more surgery and many more procedures in the days and weeks to come.

On our first day at Columbia-Presbyterian, David's new neurosurgeon, Dr. Sander Connolly, who at some time in his medical career had attended David's "Med Micro" lectures, presented me with seriously unpleasant news: David needed another operation. The knobby protrusion Dr. Hulda had been unable to dislodge at Sierta Hospital needed to be removed. I guess it was inevitable. I had to consent to a second brain surgery.

The day of David's surgery—January 17th—was another endless day of wondering, worrying, and waiting. The minute hand seemed to crawl around the clock as slowly as the hour hand. It felt as though time forgot to move. I spent the morning on a waiting room couch. We all did.

Every time a white coat or green scrubs entered the waiting room, I peered expectantly, yet hesitantly, toward the door. When the messenger was not for me, I tried to read the doctor's expression as he or she approached the patient's family. When the news was positive, the doctor's mood was airy. His or her work was successful, and he or she seemed elated. The family's anxious mood lifted as relief, then joy, spread over their faces. I smiled too as I felt their happiness. It gave me hope.

But many doctors arrived with serious looks, eyes averted, or with wait-and-see expressions. Their news was never good, and I felt sad for those families. It broke my heart to see their despair. I knew my time would come. I hoped for the airy doctor to breeze through the door towards me. Watching the interactions with the doctors and families was a lesson in emotion. Hope, joy, angst, and sorrow were etched on their faces. As I waited my turn, I knew I would be watched too.

I was eager for the news that David's surgeon would bring, yet I dreaded it too. I clung to the hope that David would be okay, but unhappy thoughts niggled in the back of my mind. They pressed toward the surface, itching to escape. I tried suppressing them, but they refused to cooperate. They haunted me. *What if David did not come back to me?* Okay, say it. Be straight! *What if he died?* I couldn't wrap my mind around that unwelcome thought. Maybe it was selfish of me, but I needed him, and I prayed for Dr. Connolly to come with a smile on his face, with a spring in his step. I wanted him to tell me happy news. Only he could end my nightmare.

When Dr. Connolly pushed through the doors, there was no spring in his step. He looked tired. He motioned me to a table across the room, and we sat. He told me that the surgery to remove the aneurysm was successful. I was relieved, but I knew there was more. Dr. Connolly explained that while David's brain was exposed, he saw a malformation of blood vessels. He called it an arteriovenous malformation (AVM), and he said it was congenital.

Though many people unwittingly have AVMs, usually they are inconsequential. With age, the risk of rupture rises, possibly leading to severe consequences, especially if the AVM is in the brain. Dr. Connolly likened the condition to a time bomb. Then he said that David needed to undergo yet another surgery—a third brain surgery—to remove the offending vessels.

Impossible! My brain was ready to explode. I made him explain it to me again and again as I drew a picture on a tiny piece of cardboard I found on the table. I still have that offending piece of cardboard—pretty bad art. Dr. Connolly told me he had to wait until the swelling in David's brain from this operation subsided and David's condition stabilized before he could perform the AVM surgery. He could not tell me when that would be. I had to wait.

When I saw David after his surgery for the removal of the aneurysm, I understood what Dr. Connolly meant. David looked destroyed. Any progress David made from the first surgery had vanished. His responses were minimal. I again coaxed him to squeeze my hand, open his eyes, or wiggle his toes—anything. I wanted a sign that he knew I was there, that he knew I loved and needed him. I may as well have been asking him to touch his elbow to his nose. David was in his own world, and that world did not include me. He was far away.

"Time," the nurses said. "You have to give him time." Time was all I had—and hope.

In a hospital, hope comes and goes like a child circling on a carousel—around and around with a wave on each pass, then quickly slipping around the curve and gone, to return soon with another wave. Like the merry-go-round, like the ebb and flow of the tide, like morning fading into night, then morning rising again, hope comes and it goes. I lived on hope. I craved the happy news days just as I dreaded those that brought sadness.

In the middle of January, soon after that second operation, a friend of ours, Dr. David Markowitz, visited. It was comforting to see him. He was the doctor who saved my life a decade earlier—but that is another story. Though I am not generally a fan of doctors, I am fond of David Markowitz. So when he stood at David's bedside in the NICU, he looked like a knight in shining armor, and my hope was briefly raised. After I recounted what happened, a story I had told several times, he presented me with another piece of paper, one with dotted lines on the bottom. I groaned.

David Markowitz is a specialist for disorders of the gastrointestinal tract. He had been summoned to perform a surgical operation called percutaneous endoscopic gastrostomy (PEG) on David. He explained that it involved inserting a tube into David's abdomen. The PEG tube would feed directly into his stomach. Since David's comatose state prohibited him from ingesting food, this was the best way to nourish him. First Dr. Markowitz would thread a flexible tube with a camera on its end through David's mouth, down his esophagus, and into his stomach. The camera would determine where in David's abdomen the incision would be made to install a port for the feeding tube.

Until now David received all nourishment via an IV bag containing nutrients. He was fed on a slow drip. Dr. Markowitz explained that, although inserting the PEG tube was considered an invasive surgery, it involved little risk and would not cause David discomfort. I knew, though, that this was a sure sign of a long recovery. David was going to be a high-paying guest of Columbia-Presbyterian Hospital for an unknown period of time. Dr. Markowitz convinced me that the procedure needed to be done. I signed.

With the PEG inserted, thick, tan-colored liquid with zero appeal flowed through the tube directly into David's stomach. Yuck! It made liver, which I abhor, look appetizing. Despite its lack of appeal, its minerals and vitamins gave David the strength to stay alive. A long time would pass before "real" food passed over his lips again, though I'm sure David's favorite bean and veggie burrito was not on his mind anyway.

A few days after the PEG insertion and less than a week after arriving at Columbia-Presbyterian, David's doctor said he would remove the endotracheal tube from David's mouth. He said it was uncomfortable for patients to have air tubes extending from their mouths for prolonged periods of time. *No kidding!*

He added that the tubes often caused additional complications. I was ecstatic that he was going to remove it. Improvement! Then he dashed my hopes with his next proclamation: he would perform a tracheotomy—a minor surgery, but surgery nonetheless. The doctor said that he would insert a tube into David's trachea, which would allow oxygen to flow directly into David's lungs.

A childhood memory surfaced of an old woman with a hole in her neck. When she held her finger over the cavity and spoke, she sounded like Darth Vader. *No! No! No!* I would not allow the doctor to cut open David's throat, to destroy his voice, to make it raspy—not his beautiful voice.

Three weeks before David's trauma, my brother John had called with news that the doctors were planning a tracheotomy on his son, who also suffered a traumatic brain injury. I felt sad. Little John was a young man! A tracheotomy would be devastating. Fortunately, Little John improved and was able to breathe independently before the doctors could wield their knives at his throat. His tracheotomy was canceled. David was not so fortunate.

Since David was unable to breath on his own, it was obvious that he needed the respirator to remain alive. I knew the tracheotomy had to be done, and I signed on the dotted line . . . again. Once more the seriousness of his trauma was impressed upon me, and it dashed my hopes of this nightmare ending anytime soon.

The tracheotomy tube was inserted. Gone was the beautiful voice on our answering machine. David's pre-trauma voice says, "I'm sorry—we don't answer our phone. Please leave a message, and we will call you back." I never erased that message, and each time our phone rang, I heard what once was. It made me happy and it made me sad. I hope I never lose David's message with his lilting voice, now recorded—a reminder of more carefree days.

Would David, with his new raspy voice, be able to deliver his lectures, discuss science with his colleagues, or direct the work of his students? I wondered how he would even talk with me.

CHAPTER 15

Emotional Roller Coaster

Despite David's operations, the days continued in a blur. It was hard to know night from day. It didn't make much difference— not for the unlucky patients bound to their beds, and not for me. I was going nowhere. The nurses came and went. They checked the dials and tubes on the machines attached to David. They added liquids to his feeding tube every few hours. Steak and potatoes it was not! No matter. David, who does not eat beef, wouldn't have eaten that anyway.

I did what I could to keep David comfortable. I kept his pillows fluffed and his blanket pulled up. I kept his legs and feet propped up too. They were encased in giant, blue boots called Ankle Contracture Boots. They looked like something Neil Armstrong wore as he stepped onto the moon. Not terribly stylish, but they helped to prevent a complication called "foot drop." When patients are expected to be bedridden for an extended period of time, which unfortunately David was going to be, weakness or even paralysis of the muscles in the foot or ankle areas may occur. To prevent this complication, David wore these boots. They helped to retain the normal tension in his feet so that he would not be forced to walk on his toes when the time came for him to rise from his bed. Even with these boots, his feet often fell to the side and needed proper support.

He didn't need another complication. So, I collected pillows and stuffed them around his feet.

The muscles of the body, especially in the arms and legs, may atrophy when a patient is bedridden for a long time. This means a patient's limbs diminish in size or strength and become weakened. David quickly dwindled in size. His slight 145-pound toned body lost mass. His legs looked skeletal. In just a few weeks, he lost between ten and twenty pounds. By the time he was released from the hospital nearly three months later, the scale registered a thirty-pound reduction. Not a recommended program for weight loss!

Jared, Kiersten, and I exercised David's arms and legs often throughout each day. Jared focused on his legs, since they were heaviest. Even with the weight loss, they felt like cement blocks. Jared repeatedly raised and lowered David's legs, bending them from his knee to his chest and rotating his ankles. Though Kiersten and I also worked on David's legs, we concentrated on his wrists, hands, and arms—rotating his wrists, bending his fingers, and rubbing his arms to increase his circulation. We kept his joints flexible.

When Kiersten and Jared returned home to their own lives, I continued exercising David's limbs. Each night before I dragged myself back to my borrowed apartment, I'd slather cream on David's legs and run my hands up and down them to stimulate his circulation and strengthen his muscle tone. It was hard not to remember those once-strong legs poking out of his running shorts, racing down the street to the parks for a multi-mile run.

Foremost among David's problems, now that the aneurysm had been clipped and removed, was the removal of the AVM time bomb in David's head. It could burst at any time. The risk of rupture increases with age, and David was *not* getting any younger. How could anyone live anxiety-free knowing a tangle of blood vessels could bleed at any time, causing stroke, neurological damage, or even death? These offending blood vessels had to go, but before they could be removed, time had to pass. David needed to regain his stamina after the previous two operations.

There was still a lot of pressure buildup in David's skull. To release the pressure, Dr. Connolly ordered an EAD (external arterial drain). He drilled a hole into David's frontal bone, which is located at the top and forward part of the head. The site was positioned about three inches above and slightly to the right of David's right eye. A tube was inserted through this hole into his skull to act as a conduit for draining the excessive fluid from David's brain, relieving the pressure and allowing his swollen brain to regain its natural shape.

Dr. Connolly scheduled the operating room for Monday, January 24th, but the pressure on David's brain was still too high. He explicitly and graphically explained that if he opened up David's skull too soon, his cerebellum could squish out. My eyes bugged out, and my jaw dropped. We agreed that David was not yet ready. The operation was postponed. More waiting.

During this time, additional surprises were in store. David's temperature rose dangerously high—a possible sign of infection. No one knew the cause of the fever or the source of any infection, but some possibilities were entertained. The doctors concluded that the probable cause was a blood clot near the central venous catheter inserted in David's jugular vein. The line had been threaded through a large vein in David's neck, called the superior vena cava, and ended at a point near his heart. It monitored various bodily functions, such as heart rate and blood pressure. It also administered medications considered too caustic to be dripped through the less invasive A-line (intra-arterial line).

The A-line is a smaller catheter usually inserted into an artery on the inner side of the wrist. It too monitored blood pressure, and it can also be used to draw blood for various lab tests or to track the oxygen concentration in the blood. The central venous catheter is generally used when a patient is expected to require intense medical care for an extended period of time. (There are those words again.) All catheters may cause infection, but David's catheter, because of the suspected blood clot, would be more apt to grow bacteria. Although the possible clot was frightening, it was better than the doctor's next suspicion: an infection in David's central nervous system, which could imply meningitis or encephalitis.

Both meningitis and encephalitis are inflammations of the membranes surrounding the brain. They are caused by viruses or bacteria, which can enter through the bloodstream. Depending on the severity of the infection and the response of treatment, patients may expect full recovery, though the process may be slow. In more severe cases, meningitis or encephalitis may cause permanent brain and nerve damage or loss of hearing or speech. They can cause seizures, loss of muscle control, and memory loss. In some cases these diseases are fatal.

I was relieved when the infections were ruled out. A blood clot near the central venous catheter was preferable. The nurses removed and replaced the catheter. Then, to help reduce the fever, they covered David with an Arctic Blanket, a cooling device.

Since the doctors also suspected David was experiencing seizures during this time, they ordered several EEGs. An EEG is a non-invasive, risk-free diagnostic procedure that can identify and evaluate neurological disorders, such as seizures, brain lesions, tumors, encephalitis, or stroke. A camera was set up in the room to monitor David's every movement. He was under constant surveillance—sort of like Big Brother from George Orwell's *1984*. Though I am generally opposed to a loss of privacy, in this case I welcomed the constant surveillance. Fortunately, each of David's EEG results was negative. Negative was good.

Not all the surprises happened to David. Mother Nature decided to "bless" me with sniffles, itchy eyes, drippy nose, and a slight cough. I guess I should have been surprised that it took so long for me to get sick. Everyone knows a hospital is *no* place to keep well. Of course, the stress, the long twelve- to fourteen-hour days in the hospital, and little sleep did not help either. The first tickle in my throat and my first sniffle nearly sent me into a panic. I knew that I shouldn't be wandering the halls of the hospital spreading germs to the unlucky inhabitants of the NICU, and I surely did not want to cause additional complications for David. I shortened my days, went to bed earlier, and got more rest, and I began wearing a surgical mask while in the NICU. I was lucky. This cold was short-lived, unlike my regular colds, which sometimes last for weeks. Perhaps my stars were aligned, which was fortunate because I couldn't stay away from David.

Yet there were more surprises. This roller coaster seemed never-ending, with its ups and downs and its left curves. On Monday, January 24th, the day the AVM operation was scheduled and canceled, David showed signs of awareness. His lethargy lifted. He responded to the doctor's commands. He even moved his right hand, which mostly rested limply at his side. I was hopeful.

My cousin Patti arrived to visit that day as she did most days. Each day was the same. Some gains. Some regressions. I always encouraged David to show off—squeeze my hand, blink his eyes, his normal repertoire. Patti and I were excited to see his unexpected alertness, which was more than he had demonstrated since his ordeal began. You might imagine our elation when Patti said goodbye to David that day, and he raised his hand and waved to her. That night Patti wrote the following email to family and friends:

I have to share a personal experience that left me teary eyed and filled with joy. As I was standing at the foot of David's bed, saying my goodbyes, much to my astonishment, he raised his left hand and waved goodbye to me. Can you believe it? It's a wave I will never forget. Who would have thought a wave could touch your heart in such a way?

Patti's email touched many hearts. David's father wrote:

It's midnight and I was about to get ready to turn in for the night. Decided to check my e-mail again and boy, am I ever glad I did! What a wonderful surprise. I should sleep well tonight.

A few days later, on January 26th, David gave his night nurse a scare, which in turn frightened me. When David's night nurse Melody checked on David in the middle of the night, she found him sitting up in bed. That's not so scary, except that David had no control over his body. He was unable to move, and his muscles were slack, but somehow he had found the bed controls that raise and lower the mattress and fiddled with them enough to bring his upper mattress to a dangerously high, perpendicular position. He was seated precariously upright—nearly flopping over like a Raggedy Andy doll. Before any harm came to David, Melody settled him back into bed with the controls safely out of reach.

When Melody, whom I absolutely adored, told me of the incident the next morning, I detected a barely perceptible grin on David's face. He had enjoyed his unwitting prank. When Melody asked him how he was that morning, he gave her the okay sign. Melody and I laughed hysterically, and I saw the edges of David's crooked lips rise even more into a slight grin. That teeniest effort of connecting index finger and thumb to make the okay sign and the slight rise of his lips were monumental. To us, who are healthy, these are minute efforts, but to David, struggling for a grasp on life, it was a milestone.

There would be many milestones over the next weeks, months, and years, and many challenges too. The next challenge facing us was David's operation for removal of the AVM. He was on the operating room schedule again, this time for Friday morning, January 28th. I prayed we'd count it as a success and a milestone.

CHAPTER 16

Third Time's a Charm

It was difficult sleeping Thursday night before David's AVM operation. I found it impossible to believe he had to endure yet another brain surgery. He had won the lottery by surviving his first operation on January 13th. He'd defied all odds when he was still breathing after his second surgery on January 17th. What were his chances of overcoming a third surgery so soon after his last one? Three brain surgeries within a month! It was too much to expect of anyone. But not having the surgery was not an option. There was no choice.

Thursday night was especially difficult too because David was agitated with me. This was the first time I had experienced this behavior. Of course, I wanted to be with him, near his bedside, but as I held his hand the night before the surgery, he twisted my fingers. He squeezed and bent them backwards. Kiersten and Jared feared he might break them. He was strong, but I didn't believe he would hurt me. Actually, I was glad to see some emotion. It seemed as though he wanted to tell me something, but I couldn't discern it. Maybe my ignorance angered him. Maybe he'd reached ample awareness to comprehend he was in the hospital. Maybe he wanted to know why. Perhaps he sensed another brain surgery, and he didn't want it. I could second-guess forever and never know his real reasons.

I felt as though I were betraying him by allowing the doctors to invade his brain again. Maybe he sensed my fear and confusion. For whatever reason, he pushed me away. He was angry. He made strong hand motions for me to leave the room—not Kiersten, not Jared, only me. That hurt! I didn't want to go, but I had to spare him the agitation. I was scared—not *of* him, but *for* him—so I left. I lingered outside the curtain, keeping vigil beyond his awareness. With me out of sight, David regained his composure. When I sensed his calmness, I returned in time to tuck him in for the night. He would need rest before his surgery.

Before I left that night, I spoke with Melody. She assured me that everything would be okay. She said she'd call if there was any change, and I gave her my cell number. She encouraged me to call if I became overly worried and insisted I call at 4:00 a.m. to be sure the surgery was on schedule. I set my clock, and I did exactly that. The surgery was happening!

While New York slept, I tossed and turned and anticipated another long day of waiting for the surgery to be over. As the sky lightened, I slipped into the shower, got dressed, and tiptoed out the door. With a heavy heart, I walked the short distance to the hospital. Though it was earlier than my usual arrival, there was an abundance of activity in David's room—prep for the operation. I stayed near but out of the way.

Around 7:00 a.m., two attendants wheeled David to the operating room. The attendants were kind and tried to calm me. I walked with them as far as I was allowed. Then I leaned over David and whispered that I would be here when he returned. I kissed him and hoped it was not for the last time. I told David I loved him. I told him I needed him and that I always would, that I could not live without him. Nothing like guilt to make him work harder to survive! He thrived on competition. Now it was time to beat all odds again. When the doors closed behind him, I stood there. I watched until the gurney was out of sight. Then I allowed the tears to escape. I didn't even bother to brush them away as I made my way to the waiting room to once again *wait*.

Dr. Connolly had told me David would not return to his room until about two or three o'clock—a full day's work for both the doctor and David—and for me. Waiting is hard, tedious work.

I remember feeling nervous in a calm sort of way. And anxious! And eager! And hopeful! Nervous that everything would go wrong. Anxious about the danger of David's surgery. Eager for Dr. Connolly's pronouncement that David would soon be better. And hopeful, mostly hopeful, that David would return home, and life would be as it was—long walks in the parks, breakfast at our favorite café on weekends, and sushi on Sunday.

So many emotions flooded in. I tried to quash the despairing thoughts—the ones in which I feared the worst. I imagined my reaction if I received the ultimate bad news: "We did everything we could, but David did not survive the operation." Or "David will never have another cognitive thought again." Or "He'll never walk or talk again." Or "He may not know you anymore." Or "I'm afraid David is in a permanent vegetative state. His brain is too damaged. We can't repair it." Every possible scenario fought for center stage in my mind. I tried to suppress them because I knew how I'd react if any were true. I would crumble. My life would end. I wouldn't want to exist— not without David, my best friend, my love.

It was hard to watch the parade of scrub-clad doctors search the waiting room for their patients' families—delivering good news or bad. I had become very adept at knowing which type of news the doctors bore based on their expressions, and I waited with hope and dread for my turn. I waited as patiently as I could until the hands of the clock passed three o'clock. Then I was no longer patient. I expected the surgery to be over by then. Dr. Connolly had said so. My mind raced into overdrive. Something was wrong. Bad news loomed. Four o'clock came. Still no news. Four-thirty! Five o'clock!

Finally Dr. Mayer, a doctor on Dr. Connolly's team, pushed through the door. His face looked reassuring. I felt a surge of relief as he said that David was okay. He apologized that the operation took longer than expected. Partially due to a delay in occupying the operation room, they started two hours late, he explained. I wish someone had thought to tell me! Dr. Mayer told me he performed an angiogram on David. An angiogram is a procedure in which a neuroradiologist inserts a catheter containing a dye or contrast into the patient's vein and threads it to the desired area. In this case, it was David's brain. An angiogram is an imaging test that allows X-rays to monitor the blood flow and helps to determine any damage to the veins. Dr. Mayer said that the angiogram confirmed that the AVM was completely removed and that everything was in order. Phew!

Dr. Mayer said Dr. Connolly was completing David's surgery and closing his skull. David would then go to recovery and remain there until he stabilized. It could be hours before he returned to his cubicle in the NICU.

I was glad that the operation was over, but I remained impatient. I couldn't wait—not a second longer. I needed to see for myself that he was okay. Every fifteen minutes, I'd poke my head through the NICU door looking for activity in David's room. Nothing! His recovery was long. Dr. Mayer was right. Hours passed, and I waited.

When David finally returned to his NICU cubicle, he was

a scary sight. He looked like he had been through a war, and I guess, in a way, he had been. He spent the day battling for his life . . . and he won! Again, he won. But not without scars. Again, time would be our healer. It would be our friend.

Shortly after this surgery, David finally emerged from his coma and I was so excited. Since he could hear and see me, I hoped our communication would improve, but it would be some time before he was completely alert.

The next days passed much like the ones before. Each day David grew stronger and slightly more aware. I was relieved no more surgeries were scheduled. Dr. Connolly finally pronounced him out of critical danger and arranged new accommodations in the Step Down Unit, which is for patients needing less intensive care.

CHAPTER 17

Phew!

The Step Down Unit was on the eighth floor. It was a four-bed room with a single nurse assigned to four patients. The room was large with a full wall of windows overlooking the Hudson River. From David's bed next to the window, the George Washington Bridge in its majestic beauty was in full view. I tried to position David so he could enjoy the view. Though no longer comatose, he was largely unaware and never seemed to notice the city beyond his window. He was in his own world, and it did not include the George Washington Bridge or me.

Although there were four beds in the room, when David arrived there was only one other occupant—an elderly man who was very vocal and determined to escape his bed. He almost made it a few times too. During David's second day in the unit, beds were needed for three more patients, and somebody's well-meaning but misguided decision had David moved to a private room.

The private room was on the general floor and overseen by the floor staff. It did not have a private nurse supervising it. In a private room David would have been helpless. He was completely unaware of himself or his surroundings. He was unable to call for help since he was intubated. He wasn't able to locate the call button, let alone push it. In fact, he couldn't even comprehend what a call button was. The man in the bed next to David was more able to handle a room on his own without constant supervision. He could move about and use the call button when needed. David could do nothing but lie there.

I appealed to Nurse Joan, David's day nurse, with whom I had become friendly. I recognized her love for her work and her dedication to her patients. Joan agreed that the decision had been unwise, saw no logic in moving David, and interceded with the powers that be. And so, thankfully, David remained under Joan's vigilant supervision for several more days.

The day when David would have to be transferred to another facility drew near. His doctors had done what they could for him and he was stable. Now it was time for recovery and rehabilitation. But it was still undecided where he would go when he was released from the hospital. It was obvious that he could not return home. He was too sick and needed constant medical care—care I was not able to provide.

A social worker encouraged me to find a rehabilitation facility for him. In fact, I was required to give her the names of three acute facilities and five subacute facilities to which David could be transferred. She said that when the doctors were ready to release him, the procedures went swiftly.

A subacute facility offers only one hour of therapy a day, and I refused to supply any names. It is essentially a stopover for patients who are not expected to improve or for those who cannot withstand a rigorous schedule of three hours of physical, occupational, and speech therapy a day. That is what is expected of patients in a high-powered acute facility and what I wanted for David. A subacute facility is a nursing home—pure and simple. It is for folks past their prime, seniors who need assisted living. It was not an option for my young, vibrant, very determined husband. (Well, he had been all of those things three weeks earlier.)

The social worker and I argued. She insisted, and I insisted right back. We each held our ground. She was doing her job. I was doing mine. Though the social worker said that I was required to provide a selection of names, she was unable to offer advice. She provided me with a list of facilities in New Jersey but admitted knowing nothing about them. New Jersey is less than two miles from the hospital. No doubt a hefty percentage of the patients at Columbia-Presbyterian are from New Jersey. There simply was no excuse for her lack of knowledge. I told her that I would not leave David's bedside, and therefore, it was impossible for me to "go shopping" for nursing homes. Though Kiersten and Jared scouted out several nursing homes in New Jersey, I refused to provide the social worker with any subacute options. I did, however, do my homework. I searched the Internet for the best acute rehabilitation hospitals in my area. Each provided the maximum hours of daily therapy and each had an outstanding reputation.

The social worker said that the acute facilities would require proof that David could withstand their rigorous schedule and would send a representative to assess his abilities. David's doctors would also need to approve his placement in an acute facility. Her goading didn't work. I stood my ground, though admittedly I wondered if David could manage the rigors of an acute hospital. He could barely raise his hand, but I insisted that he would pass their tests. He was strong. His determination in life was great. He always set his goals high, and he always met them. He would do it again. He had to!

To be sure that the scales weighed in my favor, I lobbied each of David's doctors. I cornered them one by one. I needed their assurances that David was strong enough to withstand an acute rehabilitation hospital. I bragged about how highly motivated he was, how goal-orientated he was, and how determined and strong he was before the trauma. I was shameless—but it worked! They each agreed.

Truthfully, I don't know what made them believe. David lay limply in his bed, barely able to move a muscle. He did not look motivated or determined. During the final evaluation, a team of doctors surrounded him. I watched each probe of the reflex hammer. Nothing—not even a twitch. The doctor explained that she used this tool to test David's deep tendon reflexes. I watched her face for signs of approval or disapproval. She tapped his knees, his elbows, and his fingers. I still detected no movement, and my spirits fell. He was going to fail. But then I heard "Ahhh!" and "Yes!" and "Look!"

Finally, I could stand it no longer. "What? What are you seeing?"

Though she detected abnormalities in David's central nervous system, she said there was movement deep within his tendons. They were active, and that was good. When I could wait no longer, I asked if David was a candidate for acute rehabilitation, and she said, "Most definitely!" I breathed.

David stayed at Columbia-Presbyterian for just a day past three weeks. Then, as the social worker had predicted, everything moved quickly. I chose Radburn Rehabilitation Center in New Jersey—an acute facility. It had an excellent reputation for brain trauma rehabilitation, and it was about thirty minutes from our home, without traffic. I packed David's personal belongings— massage creams, gauze bandages, bedpan, and restraining mitts. It was amazing how much stuff was moving with us. I need not have taken it. Radburn used none of it. They had their own ways of doing things, and so the stuff got stuffed in a closet—a fitting place for stuff.

It was exciting to be leaving Columbia-Presbyterian, and it was bittersweet too as I said my goodbyes to the nurses and doctors who cared so well for David . . . and me. I knew that this departure was an important step toward David's recovery, but I still did not yet know how long that recovery would take.

This time I rode in the back of the ambulance with David. It was no smoother than the ambulance that transported David and me to Sierta Hospital. Rap music blared from the radio. Do you see something wrong with this picture? Do they not teach first responders in ambulance school that they are transporting sick people—that perhaps a serene atmosphere would be more conducive to wellness? Maybe Pachelbel's "Canon" or Alex Di Grassi's "The Water Garden" or Deuter's "Sun Spirit"—any of these would have been welcome and have provided a much-needed calming effect. (In fact, these composers provided me with a sense of quietude while writing this book.)

To complicate matters, the driver couldn't find Radburn. Shouldn't the driver have used MapQuest before picking up David? It was apparent he expected me to guide him. Since I'd never been there, I wasn't much help. David's agitation grew. No wonder! The long trip and noise were enough to set anyone's nerves on edge. I too was upset, especially when the driver raced past the expressway exit. I watched with exasperation as the exit we wanted faded in the rear window. We sped down the highway in search of a U-turn.

When we finally arrived, I experienced a strange feeling as we waited for the elevator. I was relieved to be rid of the ambulance, but I was nervous of this new unknown. I wondered what this part of the adventure would present.

CHAPTER 18

Colorful Roommate

As the elevator doors opened, a team of nurses met David and his entourage. It was obvious the nurses were expecting him. They directed the paramedics down the hallway to the double doors past the nurses' station. One nurse stealthily tapped a code into a keypad, and the door slowly opened. We passed through—Jared, Kiersten, Kiersten's daughters (Treska, 9, and Kaya, 7) who had recently arrived, and me.

I soon learned that this floor was the lockdown unit. Only authorized personnel could access the door using a secret code. It was locked because it housed some seriously disturbed brain-injured patients. It didn't take long to meet the first "inmate." He was David's roommate. As the nurses settled David into his room, hooked him up to the various IVs and monitors, and completed the mounds of paperwork, I met Uncle Gino.

Uncle Gino was in his eighties at least. He was a large man with a long face topped with a bald head. He looked exactly like someone's sweet great-grandpa, but he terrified me. The television over his bed blared. For one who does not have a TV, I was unsettled by the noise, and I knew it would be troublesome for David as his awareness grew. It didn't help that Uncle Gino played with the switch for what seemed like hours, flicking it on and off and then on again for no apparent reason. He wasn't watching the TV.

The nurse attempted to settle Uncle Gino and drew his curtain closed, which provided us with pseudo privacy. But this did not deter Uncle Gino. We were his entertainment *du jour*. No sooner was the privacy curtain drawn between the beds when Uncle Gino grabbed it, pulled it aside, and stuck his very large balding head across the space. He was curious. The nurse firmly pulled the curtain back into place and just as firmly, yet gently, encouraged Uncle Gino to watch his TV. Then she left me to fend for myself.

I squeezed into the cramped space between the beds to adjust a twisted hose on David's respirator. The curtain whipped away again, and I stifled a scream as Uncle Gino nearly grabbed me. I dodged him, then edged my way down the side of David's bed, keeping as far away as possible. I never went to that side of the bed again—not when Uncle Gino was in the room.

David was oblivious. He wasn't bothered by Uncle Gino, but I freaked out. When Uncle Gino started screaming for the nurses, I nearly lost it. He pleaded to use the bathroom. He begged for what seemed to be an eternity, but no one came. At first I wasn't concerned. I knew the nurses were busy, and I figured they would tend to him in due time, but eventually it seemed as though they were ignoring him. My mind went into overdrive. If they ignored Uncle Gino, would they ignore David when he needed their help? I didn't want David to be here. Nursing home and hospital horror stories raced through my mind, and I thought we might be the main characters in one. I wanted to pack David up and take him home, but I knew that was impossible.

Instead, I calmly approached the nurses' desk and told the nurse that David's roommate needed to use the bathroom. She must have seen the horror on my face and took pity on me. She patiently explained that Uncle Gino had a condom catheter, which allowed him to void directly into a bag. He didn't need the use of a real bathroom. Though I was embarrassed, I was relieved to know that he was not being abused.

Uncle Gino had a repertoire of tricks to share with us that night. Next he began to moan, "Maria! Maria, please come. Where is Maria? Ma-ri-a, where are you? I want Maria. Maria, Maria, Maria!" His voice drifted off, then he moaned again. After thirty minutes of this repetitive behavior, my concern heightened, and I again sought out a nurse. She explained that Maria was Uncle Gino's daughter, who only visited on weekends. I felt sad. But I was sadder to know that Uncle Gino didn't understand where his daughter was.

Because of the commotion in David's room with Uncle Gino, Treska and Kaya sat in the waiting room. We feared that Uncle Gino's bizarre behavior would frighten them. The nurse reassured me that Uncle Gino was harmless and he would soon go to sleep, but I wondered how she knew. He looked overly animated to me. I later learned that each night sleeping pills were doled out like candy to all the patients. Quiet nights!

Uncle Gino's sleeping pills must have been placebos that night because they didn't work. Perhaps the excitement of his new roommate was too much for him. I know the excitement of Uncle Gino was over the top for me. For the first time, I broke down and cried shamelessly in front of nurses. I begged them to change David's room, but there were no empty rooms. We were stuck. They did promise to move David when a room became available—tomorrow, the day after, next week.

I was inconsolable. Terrance, David's charge nurse, felt for me—either that or he feared I was ready to flip out. Then he would need another bed. He promised he'd try to find a room.

In the meantime, he wheeled Uncle Gino to the small waiting room down the hall. I was horrified when I saw him strap Uncle Gino to his wheelchair. *How cruel!* I thought. I didn't know then that it was protocol and routinely done for the safety of the patients. I felt guilty. Because of me, Uncle Gino was ousted from *his* room and banished to the waiting room. My heart broke when Uncle Gino cried and pleaded to return to his room to go to bed. The nurses assured me that he was fine and that, if he went to bed, he would soon ask to get up. This was typical behavior for him, they said. Though I was not comforted, my selfish self was glad he was gone.

Finally, David was settled in, and Kiersten joined her daughters in the waiting room. What a surprise she found! Treska and Kaya were engaged in a lively conversation with Uncle Gino. In our angst over David's situation, it hadn't occurred to us that when we were relieved of Uncle Gino's presence, he would be keeping company with Treska and Kaya. Kiersten laughed as she told me that her girls were delighted by him. They only saw a very old grandfather—though Treska did later confess he seemed somewhat strange. Treska and Kaya's acceptance of this strange man with his odd behaviors makes me smile. The wonders of children!

I wasn't comfortable leaving David in this strange place, not even for a single night. I was confused, frightened, and exhausted. I couldn't imagine how David felt. But I had no choice. It was late. The girls needed to go to bed, and I had the only car. When Jared volunteered to stay the night with David and the nurse wheeled a sleeping chair into the room for him, I was relieved.

With heavy heart, I went home for the first time in more than three weeks to the scene of the trauma. I didn't want to see the black marks made so carelessly by the paramedics as they bounced David's gurney into the freshly painted walls. I was nervous entering our bedroom, where the nightmare began. Images of David writhing on the bed in pain played across my mind. I was hesitant to sleep in our bed—so big and so empty without David by my side. And I was worried that David was apprehensive too. These unwelcome thoughts tumbled around my mind as I drove home. As we approached the gate to our complex, my phone rang. It startled me. It was Jared. I expected bad news. I expected him to tell me to return to the hospital, so I was relieved when he said that David was sleeping peacefully in a room across the hall. Thank you, Terrance! Now I could sleep too.

The next morning, I arrived early—eager to see David's new room situation. I found David down the hall in a much smaller room, a closet almost. I crawled over chairs to get to his bed next to the window, but still this was far better. It was calm.

David's new roommate, Ray, another recent survivor of traumatic brain injury, was quiet and subdued. His wife, Nancy, assured me that even without the brain injury, Ray was a gentle man. She told me her husband was a professor, and I felt an immediate kinship with her. Ray taught accounting at a local New Jersey college, and he had his own accounting firm. He was a big, handsome man with a beautiful wife and three lovely daughters.

I was pleased when the nursing staff moved both Ray and David to Uncle Gino's much larger room and moved Uncle Gino to the smaller room. Though I was grateful, guilt flooded me again. I was the cause of uprooting Uncle Gino once more. The nurses assured me that Uncle Gino was not fazed by the change, and I was relieved.

Soon I met each of Ray's daughters (Janis, Celia, and Ellen) and their families, and I knew this move was a good decision.

The larger room would accommodate our families more easily, and even with many visitors, it would not be as chaotic as living with Uncle Gino. It was pleasant, and I felt safe walking between the beds.

Living in the confined space of a hospital room with two beds and little moving space was an interesting new adventure. Ray in the bed next to David with Nancy and their three daughters fussing about him was a welcome diversion. It was impossible not to hear their conversations. Though I tried to give them privacy and politely averted my eyes, I knew what was going on in their corner of the room, just as they must have known what was going on in mine. After all, we were living together in what seemed like a closet.

While our husbands slept, Nancy and I shared stories. It was the start of my second healing. My first healing began when I met Judy Thau at Columbia-Presbyterian with her husband, Steve, who was only a few cubicles away from David in the NICU. Judy, Nancy, and I were thrown into this abyss called TBI, and each of us was trying to crawl out of it in her own way. No matter how much we wished or hoped or prayed, nothing could change the nightmare we were all trapped in. It was good for David to have Ray as a roommate. It was good to have Nancy as my confidant. Sadly, it lasted only for a week.

When Nancy told me that Ray had to return to the hospital for another surgery on his brain, I didn't know if I would ever see them again. Nancy and I exchanged email addresses—our link to each other's world—and promised to keep in touch. Although Nancy expected Ray to return to Radburn, it was doubtful that David and Ray would be roommates again. Beds on the brain-injured ward were in demand. Empty beds were filled almost before the linens were changed.

And so it was. As a clean sheet was slipped on Ray's just-vacated bed, the blankets pulled up, and the pillows fluffed, another patient was rolled in. David's new roommate was Avi. He arrived with an entourage of family members—his father Simon, his mother Rebekah, and his wife Rivka.

Avi was a young man—thirty-one. I was sad for his family. Avi was the father of a boy and two girls—all under the age of four. *How did this happen to such a young man? How unfair!* The unfairness of David's injury was present in my mind too. Useless thoughts, they were.

After the flurry of activity and while Avi and David slept as calmly as anyone with a brain injury can sleep, Rebekah, Simon, and I started the process of getting to know each other. It was good to have someone to talk with—someone who was also bumping down the highway of brain injury. They were kind people, and they were devoted to their son. It was reassuring to know that either Rebekah or Simon would be at the hospital twenty-four hours a day, seven days a week. Avi would never be alone. When I left for home each night for much-needed rest and to tackle household chores, I was comforted knowing that David would not be alone. It allowed me to sleep at night.

And so, we settled in at Radburn, this next phase in recovery for David. I didn't know of the changes to come, but for now, we were as comfortable as anyone could be in a lockdown unit housing seriously brain-injured patients.

CHAPTER 19

Befriending the Staff

Who would have thought that Radburn would become home? When we arrived on the evening of February 7th, my life was vague. Unlike my normal structured life, hospital life caused me to become disoriented. I didn't know what to expect from moment to moment. Normally I had a routine. I would rise at 5:50 each morning, drive about fifty minutes to school, and teach my six- and seven-year-old "kiddles." I would show them how to read, how to string words together to form sentences, and how to join those sentences to make paragraphs. Throw in math, science, and social studies, some handwriting, music, and art, and then I would return home to run errands (getting gas, picking up books at the library, popping into the grocery store to grab something for dinner, etc.). Once home, I might fix a salad, wrap bean burritos, or as David often said, "Make something simple." He wasn't picky, but to me, nothing in the kitchen is simple.

After dinner, David and I usually went for our evening "walk-talk," during which I did most of the talking. Then I'd spend the rest of the evening preparing lessons, working on my computer, writing email, revising a picture book project, or preparing my next book review. My life was crazy, but at least it was normal-crazy. This new life was abnormal-crazy. I lived day to day, and nothing seemed real. My familiar routine was gone, and my life was as upended as David's was. Life swirled around me, but I didn't feel it. I floundered in a fog.

When we arrived at Radburn, I never dreamed that we would spend the next two months of our lives there. I had no idea what our time frame would be. Nobody did. Not David's doctors, his nurses, or his therapists. Nor would they venture to guess how long David would be there, how long it would take for him to get better—or even *if* he would get better.

I immediately set out to befriend the nurses, aides, therapists, and the other patients and their families. I met many remarkable people. The nursing staff was kind and experienced—well, all but one, but that's another chapter. But it was the nursing aides who did the messy work and who were the ones I counted on for David's daily comforts.

The first aide I met was Comfort. How Comfort's Jamaican mother knew that someday her daughter's name would fit her so aptly is a mystery to me. When Comfort first walked into the room with a warm smile on her face and gazed at David, she said decisively, "He going to be better." I scrunched my forehead. I couldn't understand her strong Jamaican accent, so she said again, "He going to be better."

I looked skeptical but felt hopeful. "How do you know?"

"I just do!" she said. "I know."

Comfort uttered those words often during David's confinement. I don't know what Comfort knew or if she knew anything, but I appreciated her promise and was grateful for her belief. I wanted to believe too.

Then there were Tracie and Artrese. We connected immediately. I don't know why. We just did. I was glad when they were assigned as David's aides. Each time they entered his room, they'd ask, "How you doing, Doc?" respecting David's title. Sometimes David would nod. Most times he was unaware and remained silent. But Tracie, Artrese, and I talked. We talked while they made beds. We talked while they moved David to his wheelchair, tied his shoes, and readied him for therapy. We talked while they took care of his most personal hygiene. Tracie and Artrese took extra special care of David. They took care of me too, and I looked forward to my daily hugs with them. We hugged often, as if we hadn't seen each other in months instead of hours. Tracie and Artrese were special. They were my world. Even when Tracie or Artrese were not assigned to David, they checked on him. They checked on me too.

There were also Betty and Marie—soft-spoken and efficient. They also called David Doc and cared for him tenderly. Dorothy, Noreen, and Eugenie seemed as if they had been at Radburn forever, and they were sturdy women I relied on. I learned about their children and their grandchildren, and they learned about mine. I laughed with Cassie and Patty with their long, black braids—twenty or thirty of them clustered over their heads. It felt good to laugh with them.

Most of the aides were women, but there were a few males too. Richard was tall, dark, and handsome—the quiet type. He was a real "gentle man." David preferred him, and I relied on Richard to ready David for the night. Richard sponge-bathed David and dressed him in pajamas, all the while soothing him with his warm Jamaican voice.

The early evening hours are often the most difficult time for patients with brain damage. Like patients who suffer from dementia or Alzheimer's Disease, brain-injured patients may be affected by a state called "sundowning." Sundowning occurs near the end of the day. Patients sometimes become confused or agitated. They may appear restless, less cooperative, or anxious. No one yet knows what causes sundowning, but scientists believe it can be brought on by increased fatigue, change in schedule, or lack of a comforting environment.

David was clearly affected by this phenomenon. I could set a clock by him. As day edged into night and the sun set, like an errant child, David thrashed in his bed, made guttural sounds, and was inconsolable. It was almost as if he were trying to crawl out of his skin. I wanted to crawl out of mine too, but not for the same reasons. I was distressed by my inadequacy to comfort my husband. Nothing I said or did consoled him. The comforts I provided him during the day were useless—holding his hand or rubbing his arms did nothing but cause more agitation. Calming or encouraging words were ignored. That's when I'd call Richard. Though Richard's strong island accent was difficult for me to understand, David seemed relaxed and reassured with him. Richard calmed David and that calmed me.

Though I only mention a few of the aides, there were many, many more. There were three shifts of aides, and I'll never forget their loving care for David and me. I understand it was their job, but they gave much more. Many became friends.

The therapists too were like friends, and David spent countless hours with them while he was a "guest" at Radburn. He endured three hours of rigorous therapy each day, except weekends. His schedule was as intense as I had expected, and though it was unbearably difficult for David to exercise so long each day when he could barely move, he had to. The social worker at Columbia-Presbyterian had little hope that David would be able to do it, but I believed. David was meeting the challenge. This was a battle we would win.

Together we'd fight to regain his life—to regain mine too. It wouldn't be easy. I was David's cheerleader, though I didn't wear the white blouse and red-pleated wool skirt and bobby socks I wore as a twelve-year-old cheerleader. There was no screaming or stomping or clapping with my squad, as I did when I cheered Michael, Jimmy, or Gary on to victory on the basketball court at Blessed Sacrament Elementary School in Erie. "Jimmy, Jimmy, he's my man. If Jimmy can't do it, *no* one can!" I chanted with my squad. And with skill and a lot of luck, Jimmy would flip the basketball into the hoop. Two points!

No, my cheering with David was calm as I urged, encouraged, and sometimes goaded him in a quiet, determined manner. "Come on, David, you can do it!" "We'll do it together!" "I'll help you!" My whispered refrains translated to "David, David, he's my man. If David can't do it, *no* one can!" Two points! And another two points! And another and another! On and on and on toward recovery. My cheering would count. It was as exciting to cheer for David as it was for a twelve-year-old to win the battles on the basketball court, but it also would be life-restoring to "win" the battle of daily living on the brain-injured ward.

I could push David's wheelchair myself, and I refused to waste a single second of those one hundred and eighty minutes of therapy. As the time approached, I'd have him ready at the door. But David was helpless, and I needed an aide to assist me in getting him into the wheelchair. David was unable to put on his shoes, let alone tie them. Frankly, he probably didn't know what shoes were or even what feet were, for that matter. He had scant awareness of his world. Either I or his aide would stuff his feet into his sneakers and lace them.

Then his aide would lift David from his bed and settle him into his wheelchair. I marveled at how easily she "man-handled" him. I tried too but I couldn't safely lift him—not yet. David is not a large man, and his illness had robbed him of at least thirty pounds. Though he weighed little more than one hundred and twenty pounds and looked skeletal, he felt like dead weight. It was amazing to see the aides move big, burly men of two hundred and fifty pounds. They made it look easy. Eventually the aides trained me. There is a technique to prevent you from hurting yourself or your patient. In time and with practice, I was able to move David from bed to wheelchair and back again, though it was not an easy task. My respect for the aides grew. Their work was hard and physical.

Once David was strapped in his wheelchair, I'd push him to the gym where either Mike or Jeff met him. Mike was David's occupational therapist, Jeff his physical therapist.

Mike worked with David on fine motor skills, like putting square pegs into round holes. At times it probably seemed like that to David. The tasks looked simple. They weren't difficult for me, and they wouldn't be difficult for you or for anyone not suffering from a traumatic brain injury or a neuro- or muscular disease. In fact, they probably weren't even too challenging for a twenty-four-month-old toddler. But watching David's intense concentration as he attempted to pick up a small cube and place it into a bowl, or as he steadied a pencil long enough to circle words on a piece of paper, or as he tried to click a button on a keyboard to catch a falling ball on a computer screen before it disappeared into oblivion brought tears to my eyes many times. As I leaned against the gym door, I'd silently brush my tears away and wonder, *How has my vibrant, so smart husband been reduced to this—stacking little rubber cubes one on top of the other?*

When David finished stacking cubes, it was time for physical therapy with Jeff. Jeff worked to strengthen David's large motor muscles. I watched as David batted a large blue balloon back and forth with Jeff. What a sad scene. If the balloon had been bopped by one of our granddaughters, I wouldn't have been distressed. No, then I would have laughed when David missed the balloon as Treska or Kaya giggled in delight. But again tears escaped as I witnessed David's struggle to connect with the balloon.

My mind wandered back in time to a beach party at Lake Erie, when David, eighteen, spiked the volleyball across the net with ease. I remembered him playing squash or handball or racquetball with Phil or Saul or Woody. When I asked how he had done, he'd always humbly say that he'd won or maybe that he just barely lost. Quick on his feet, always balanced, and competent with both hands in sports, David was naturally athletic and competitive.

Now making contact with a balloon a hundred times the size of a small handball was difficult for him. And again those darn pesky tears made their way down my cheeks as I wondered, *How could my athletic, so coordinated husband be reduced to this — bopping a balloon back and forth with an adult?*

Technically the gym was off limits to anyone but patients and their therapists. A sign stating "Patients only beyond this point" was prominently posted on the door to ensure patient privacy, but it was also there to discourage family members from meddling with their loved one's therapy. I never meddled, and neither Jeff nor Mike ever shooed me away as I leaned on the wall at the far edge of the gym, watching.

There was one set of meddling parents for whom I am sure the sign was intended. Rebekah and Simon accompanied Avi into the gym, told the therapists what he could and could not do, and constantly interfered with his therapy—that is, if they allowed Avi to go to the gym at all. Rebekah and Simon made excuses for Avi. There was the delay tactic. "Avi's sleeping." Or "Can he go later?" I shook my head in wonder. Didn't they realize the hospital was full of patients and a schedule must be kept to accommodate everyone? Then there was the cancel mode. "Avi is too tired today." Or "Avi has visitors." They offered a menu of excuses, and Avi remained in bed. They were good, doting parents who meant well. But didn't they understand that Avi wouldn't get better without therapy?

They babied their son. It's understandable. Avi was hurt. Protecting him was natural. Your child, no matter how old, remains your child. Although David was not my child, I wanted to baby him too. I longed to make life easier for him, but I knew coddling would not have helped him. I refused to lower my expectations of David. His recovery depended on the effort he exerted. I would make no excuses for him!

Maybe it was that attitude that secured me an invitation into the gym. When Jeff saw my excitement over David's accomplishments, he encouraged my participation. Soon I was on the mat with David, watching as Jeff coaxed David's large muscles into action.

I particularly liked when David walked on the treadmill, which was no easy feat because David's body was like a large rag doll. Without support, his bones would collapse in a heap on the floor. So as David hung onto the rails, Jeff secured him in a harness, which was attached to a bar extending high above the treadmill. It supported much of David's weight while allowing his legs to walk on the treadmill to simulate ambulation. The contraption reminded me much of the four-wheeled baby bouncer I secured my daughter in when she was about one year old. With her feet barely touching the floor, she "walked" and bounced around the room. I guess if David raised his feet, he would have experienced the same sensation. Fortunately, his feet remained grounded as Jeff put the treadmill into action. David walked about five to ten minutes—his stamina growing longer each session.

Jeff also introduced David to the walker—the kind you might see an eighty-nine-year-old person use. David's slight, bent frame looked much like the body of an old man shuffling through life, barely erect and tottering from side to side. His fists clenched the grips and his chin grazed his chest as Jeff guided him down the hallway. I trailed behind. Jeff urged David to keep his chin parallel with the floor, but despite constant reminders, David's chin soon fell to his chest again and again. His neck muscles were simply not strong enough to support his head.

I was grateful to be accepted into the gym, to be a part of David's therapy and recovery, and to share in his progress with Mike and Jeff.

CHAPTER 20

Catching Up

Though my days at the hospital were long—between twelve to fourteen hours each day—so were my evenings at home. I spent the lonely evening hours composing email updates detailing David's condition. Our family and friends eagerly awaited these. I was their only connection to David.

At first, the email list consisted of about ten addresses of close family members. As time passed, extended family members were added, and the list grew. It grew even larger as I received email wishes from old friends from as long ago as David's high school days. Fraternity brothers from Pitt sent their wishes. Professor advisors from Rochester and San Diego; graduate student friends from Louisville and Chicago; and former students from New Orleans; Passaic, New Jersey; and Annandale-on-Hudson, New York, to name a few, wrote to express their wishes for a speedy recovery. The number of email addresses grew to more than one hundred and sixty. Word traveled fast, especially with computer technology.

Though the good wishes and encouraging sentiments were welcome, it was nearly impossible to respond to each outreach of goodwill or plea for information on David's progress, so I started the "David Updates." The updates reminded me of those end-of-the-year letters many folks write and include with their Christmas cards. I didn't particularly care for the impersonal nature of my updates, but I understood. My updates were the most efficient way to keep so many people informed about David's progress.

Each evening was also devoted to snail mail and bills. The bills overwhelmed me. They needed to be paid, and I hadn't a clue about what to do. David used to run the money part of our household. I cooked. Dealing with the mail was challenging because I couldn't discern between real mail and junk mail. I was forced to open each piece and read it several times so I wouldn't toss away something important. Of course, as a novice, even the junk mail seemed to be important. My cousin-in-law Bryce clued me in. He pointed out key phrases like "Congratulations on your good credit report. You have been selected to . . ." or "With rates as low as 7.99%, you must hurry to apply for . . ." "Toss them!" he emphatically said, but it took time for me to trust his good advice. Finally, I began pitching them with ease into the "round file" after only one reading. Now, I'm a pro. A single glance at the envelope and I know—recycle!

Next I had to set up an organizational system to pay the bills and to keep track of which bills I paid and when I paid them. I needed a filing system for easy reference. My brother John shared his system with me. My sister Suzanne tried too, but nothing worked for me. It took night after frustrating night before I finally devised a system that made sense to me. I set up a spreadsheet for each bill with the name of the company, how much the bill was for, when the bill was due, and the date on which I paid it. I paid most of the bills online. Before all the kinks were worked out of my system, I mistakenly paid several bills more than once and had to backtrack to receive credit for them.

Because of this uncertainty, I had backup systems. I took screen captures of each transaction. I had online folders to keep each of the documents, as well as paper files. I was compulsive because the bills intimidated me. Finally, I devised a system that worked, and I still use it. Before I worked this system out, I was lost. Totally lost!

CHAPTER 21

"Don't Worry" Means "Worry"

I wasn't entirely comfortable leaving David at night since he was unable to speak or use the call button if he were in trouble. It seemed dangerous. The nurses repeatedly assured me that they would check David often. Avi's parents were there too, so I developed a sense of security. When my home phone rang on February 27th as I was half out the door, I suspected my security bubble was about to burst. David and I rarely answered our landline phone. Most of the calls were from marketers, who quickly hung up when they heard David's message. I always screened the messages, so I stopped before I closed the door and listened. My skin prickled as I heard a familiar voice. Dr. Bradofsky from Radburn was leaving a message. He said not to worry—everything was okay, which, of course, meant I *would* worry and that everything was *not* okay. Doctors rarely call with good news. I dashed up the stairs, snatched the phone from the cradle, and identified myself.

Dr. Bradofsky said that David had fallen out of bed and landed on his head! Though it didn't appear to be serious, he expected a large goose egg on David's right temple. He said he would observe him. He also had arranged for an ambulance to transport David to an imaging facility the following day for a

CT scan to rule out additional trauma. I "calmly" accepted his news, told him I was on my way, and hung up.

About half way to the hospital, I lost it. I was terrified this "bump on the head" would cause more brain injury. I pounded the steering wheel and screamed, "Why? Why? How could this happen? *Why!*" as I wiped the nonstop flow of tears from my eyes. I could not get to the hospital fast enough and prayed that the expressway would be rid of its usual overwhelming commuter traffic that morning. I underwent a minor breakdown. By the time I reached the hospital, I was composed and ready to handle the situation.

When I entered David's room, he looked sheepish. I knew that look. It was a guilty look I remembered from long ago when I arrived at another hospital—a small hospital in Goshen, New York, after he had totaled his motorcycle.

Every Sunday morning in the '80s, David took his motorcycle out for about three hours—riding the winding country roads of the Catskill Mountains in New York. It was his way to relax, to ease some of the stress of the past sixty-hour workweek. That morning, however, someone had spilled oil over the surface of the road. When David's bike rounded the bend, his tires lost their grip in the oil. While his bike was hurled under an oncoming car, David was luckily thrown to the side of the road. He suffered gravel burns over his hands and arms. Had he not been wearing a full-face helmet, his chin and forehead would have been eroded. The chin bar on his helmet was!

When I arrived at the Goshen hospital, David was standing at the end of a long hallway. He turned when he heard my footsteps, and a guilty grin spread across his face. I was so grateful to see him that I simply threw my arms around him. I sensed that same feeling as I saw David's sheepish grin and the goose egg on his temple that morning at Radburn. What was he thinking? Why had he tried to get out of bed? Of course, he wasn't able to tell me.

With his trach in place, he couldn't talk. He couldn't walk either, let alone stand, but apparently that hadn't registered in his addled brain. So, when he crawled over the bedrail—no easy task—he crumpled like a rag doll and landed on his head. I could only imagine what had happened to the IV pole, which was attached via a long tube to the PEG tube in his stomach, or to the trach tube connecting his airway to the respirator. Nobody offered the information, and I didn't ask.

Several weeks after the trach was removed, David told me why he climbed out of bed. He very seriously explained that he had to meet Angeli and Mike at Bizen and that he was late. Bizen is a sushi restaurant in Great Barrington, Massachusetts. The food is good. We often went there while staying at Mike and Angeli's Berkshire home. Sometimes we met other drivers from the Lime Rock Park racetrack for dinner. On the way to the restaurant, Angeli would always sing, "Bizen's the reason! Bizen's the reason!" What she meant is Bizen was the reason to go out to dinner after a long, tiring, but exhilarating day at the track.

I was thinking "Bizen's the reason" that David ended up with a goose egg on his head and for another adventurous ambulance ride (this one for a CT scan). I couldn't help but wonder what he was thinking.

Luckily, the CT scan showed no injury from the fall, but I questioned what psychological damage the ambulance ride may have caused! Ambulance rides were like a recurring bad dream. Though the driver and the attendant were different from those who transported David from Columbia-Presbyterian to Radburn, they could have been clones. Again, loud music blared. The driver and the attendant, with voices raised, debated how to get to the imaging facility. There were wrong turns, turning around in parking lots, and retracing miles. We were lost again! David became agitated. His nurse, Terrance, tried to calm him, as I frantically peered out the back window looking for an address.

Finally, we arrived, but when I saw the waiting room, I winced. It was full. David couldn't wait. His agitation was worsening. The nurses realized this too, and they immediately whisked him back to be scanned. Thankfully the scanning room was quiet and calm. The serenity was welcome. The ambulance trip back was as chaotic as our ride to the imaging facility. The only difference was that we didn't get lost. This time I knew the way.

David's caper added consequences to his life at Radburn. The nurses outfitted him with a restraining jacket, called a Posey after the inventor John T. Posey. It was ugly—blue and white plaid. It did its job well, but it was hot and uncomfortable. Though I agreed that the restraint was necessary, I wished Radburn had used the wrist bindings that I had brought from Columbia-Presbyterian. They were less restrictive while still providing the necessary safety, and they were undoubtedly more comfortable than the jacket. I offered them, but, because of policy and maybe insurance issues, the nurses refused.

I knew David didn't understand his newly imposed limitations. I was certain he would attempt another escape, and so the straps attached to the Posey were securely tied to the understructure of his bed. It allowed him ample movement, but it also made certain that he would remain in bed.

David also had to wear giant mitts on his hands when he was alone, making it impossible for him to grasp anything. They looked like boxing gloves made of a soft, white cloth. They were cumbersome, made his hands sweat, and seemed cruel, but they were necessary. As David's awareness grew, he became a danger to himself. More than once, he attempted to pull out his trach. When I was with him, I would distract him so he wouldn't do anything to harm himself, but when I wasn't with him, I worried he might. The mitts and the Posey helped to keep him safe, but my heart broke to see him constrained.

Each morning when I arrived, David waved his mitt-enclosed hands wildly in the air at me. *What a nice greeting!* I thought the first time I saw this assumed sign of affection. Then he began grunting at me too, and I soon realized his desperation. I threw my coat off and quickly released him from the mitts and the restraining straps of the Posey.

I had planned to return to work once David was settled into the Radburn routine. Each day was filled with three hours of therapy, and he slept much of the rest of the day, so I figured he wouldn't miss me. I knew my first graders had missed me, and I longed to see them. I'd been gone from school for more than a month, and I didn't want to take advantage of my principal's generosity. Besides, I thought I could juggle both of these intense schedules.

I made a plan. If I left school at 4:00 p.m. and drove to Radburn (about an hour drive), I could spend about five hours with David each day. Those plans vanished the day that David fell out of bed—the day the restraining jacket and "boxing" gloves became a part of his life. I'd never leave him tied up in a hospital—not for my love of teaching nor for my love of my students, though I missed them desperately. So, I called my principal, Karen Bennett, to explain the new developments. She was sympathetic and spoke with the superintendent. It was settled. I was put on indefinite leave.

I didn't know when things would improve, but I did know that I'd continue my twelve- to fourteen-hour vigil with David each day. It was a good thing I did. Another misadventure occurred that made me question if I could ever safely leave David without my always watching.

About two weeks into our stay at Radburn, the nurses removed David's Foley catheter, which was inserted through his penis directly into his bladder. It allowed his urine to flow through the tube into a bag outside his body since his bladder was malfunctioning. The removal of the catheter indicated that the doctor believed that David's bladder was now working properly and that he was able to urinate on his own. It was a huge improvement, and it was exciting.

The Foley catheter was replaced with a condom catheter, which was less invasive. His urine could flow naturally from his bladder, through his penis, and into the condom catheter tube, which would empty into a bag hanging over the edge of his bed. I was thrilled that he was being weaned off the Foley catheter. It was a major step toward his regaining his health. But the condom catheter didn't last long. It didn't work for David. I suspected his body was not really ready. So, the Foley catheter was reinserted with no definite plans for removal.

One morning I found David extremely agitated. He was pressing his belly and moaning. I called his nurse, Barbara, who discovered that his urine bag was full. She used a Doppler ultrasound instrument to scan his bladder to measure the accumulated urine. It was more than 650 cc—way too much. This should never have happened. She looked sheepish as she quickly emptied the bag. It was completely full and was backing up into David's bladder. Four hundred cc is the upper level of a safe limit. More than that may cause the bladder walls to stretch, hampering bladder retraining. It may also cause urinary infections. No wonder David was in pain! He was 250 cc beyond the safe range.

How could no one have noticed his full bag? I was upset about Barbara's inept nursing care and should have reported her to the doctor or head nurse, but I didn't. Barbara was new to Radburn, and I didn't want to cause her any problems. She apologized as she changed the bag. David's problem seemed to be resolved, and nothing could change the outcome anyway. I let it pass.

About a week later, Barbara was David's nurse again. I was surprised when she told me the cheerful news that the Foley had once again been removed and a condom catheter had been attached. Usually I knew in advance of major changes, and no one had mentioned this to me. I also thought that it was strange because normally a change such as this did not occur in the middle of the night, but I was happy that the doctor thought David was well enough to try again, and I accepted Barbara's news with joy.

Barbara and I chatted while she performed her morning routines. She checked David's respirator, hung another bag of nutrients on his IV pole, and began to clean the wound around his PEG tube. Suddenly, with no explanation, she hurried out of the room, leaving David's belly exposed. There was no dressing on the wound, and the PEG tube was uncapped, leaving David's stomach vulnerable to outside germs and possible infection. I thought her actions were strange, but I also thought perhaps she'd gone to retrieve some equipment or medication to complete the dressing. When she didn't return promptly, I rationalized that she was delayed with another patient. I gently pulled David's shirt over the opening leading directly to his stomach to avoid any contamination. Moments later, I saw a wetness spreading across his shirt.

To my horror, David's stomach fluids were leaking out. I freaked out. Terrance, David's other nurse, was at Avi's bed, and I sought his help. When he saw the uncapped PEG tube and stomach fluids on David's belly, his shock was obvious. He quickly cleaned the tube and dressed the wound. That's when I noticed that David's urine bag was again full to capacity. I lifted his blanket to check the connection only to find that there was, in fact, no condom catheter. The Foley catheter had never been removed as Barbara had said. It was intact and would be so for several more weeks.

Barbara's incompetence was beyond comprehension. She had clearly told me that the condom catheter had again replaced the Foley catheter. How could she have made the same serious error twice? David was her patient. His life was in her hands. It's common practice for nurses ending their shifts to discuss each patient's progress and needs with the incoming nursing staff, so I'm certain that Barbara was apprised of David's current situation.

When Barbara returned, instead of acknowledging her mistake, she attempted to explain away the confusion with the catheter. She made excuses for David's urine bag being full. She said it was the aide's fault because it was the aide's responsibility to drain the bag. She even tried blaming it on David, complaining that he filled up his bag too fast. Then she offered a solution. She'd post a sign over David's bed reminding the staff to change his bag more often.

I would have none of it. These were routine nursing duties. None of these problems occurred on any other nursing shift. I told her that she needed to take more care with her patients. I said there was no excuse for leaving David's PEG tube uncapped. She tried to answer my rebuffs, but I cut her off. I would accept no excuses about David's care. She left in a huff.

Terrance stood quietly by watching and listening. Soon Lolly, the nurse manager, arrived. I told her that I no longer wanted

Barbara assigned to David. Lolly agreed. She knew of Barbara's first incident, and she immediately removed her from David's care. It was awkward whenever Barbara and I passed in the hallways, and we did that a lot, but we averted our eyes and ignored each other. After a time, we exchanged polite greetings, but Barbara was never again David's nurse.

CHAPTER 22

"I Love You!"

It was weird living in a hospital for twelve to fourteen hours a day. I never left—not even to go outside for a breath of air. To do so would have meant strapping David to his bed. Even when I had to use the restroom, I timed my trip to correspond with David's therapy. Occasionally I'd need to leave his room. I'd slip next to David's bed, talking to distract him, and tie the straps of his Posey to the bars beneath his bed. Though I tried to do it covertly, David recently told me that he knew what I was doing. As David was confined to bed, I was confined to his hospital room.

One thing I know about myself is that I can never be idle. I'm always working on projects. I especially needed to be busy during that time—to flood my mind with "stuff" so that I could avoid thinking. Thinking deeply about David's plight would have been unbearable, which in turn would have made me miserable. I would have resented the horror that had happened to us. Us! Even though David alone must suffer the bodily trauma, the emotional trauma had befallen us both. If I had permitted myself to think about our future, or lack of it, I know I may have become resentful and depressed. I longed for our perfect life to be returned to us. I wished, somehow, that I were able to turn back the hands of the clock on that fateful morning of January 13th. And I questioned. If only David had awakened late that morning and hadn't had time to do his exercises, if only he had done only twelve chin-ups instead of the hated thirteen—would he have been okay? Would our lives have remained the same? Even now, my questions remain unanswered, and they haunt me daily.

The doctors said that David had harbored a time bomb in his head. They said the bleed (subarachnoid hemorrhage) could have happened at any time. I can't help but wish that it had waited until David was eighty or ninety years old. Later would have been better. The TBI would not have stripped David of his relative youth and ripped away our lives. He was in his prime—a respected Columbia professor, internationally known in his field of molecular biology.

But his brain did bleed, and I was grateful that David had been home and that I too had been home. Other scenarios would have presented more dire outcomes. I couldn't even think about how he might have been driving on the highway to Columbia or how he might have been alone in his lab before his students arrived. Both of these imply a deadly outcome or more serious complications. So when I examined the other possibilities, I knew we had been fortunate.

Whenever I felt sad about our situation—and I did often enough—I reminded myself of my pleas to each doctor who performed a surgery on David. "I don't care how you give him back to me," I'd beg, "just give him back." I am thankful each day that David fought the odds to stay with me and that he continues to live and breathe and seize his life. And I am grateful to his doctors for doing their jobs well.

I brought my laptop to David's room each day. When David slept, which he did often, I'd work on my book reviews for my column Teacher's Pets on Smartwriters.com. My editor said not to worry about them and definitely not to stress over the deadlines, but knowing I had work to do and a responsibility for completing the reviews kept my mind in the present. It prevented me from playing the "What if?" game. *What if I hadn't been home to call the ambulance? What if his first surgery had been unsuccessful, as predicted — or the second or the third? What if? What if?* The what ifs can go on endlessly, and they do no good at all. Asking what if would not change my reality. My work kept my mind from drifting to places that were too dark. It kept me from dwelling on what was no more. It kept me focused and in the present, with hope for the future.

I tried to keep current with my email, which was overflowing and kept me overly busy. Since my evenings had so few hours, I began to write the "David Updates" during the day while David slept. Family and friends eagerly awaited these missives to follow his progress.

I wrote about each tiny accomplishment. I rarely wrote about the failures, the problems, or my fears. I shared only gains—offering hope, conveying only that David was getting better. I needed to believe that.

Looking back, I wonder if that was fair—fair to David, fair to our family and friends, or more importantly, fair to me. I think I focused on David's achievements because, to me, they meant that he was getting better. I knew if I acknowledged his failures, his lack of substantial improvement, I couldn't sustain the strength I'd need to weather his trauma.

Then on March 1st . . . a milestone! David could breathe completely on his own and his trach was removed. I finally heard the much-coveted words "I love you!" Words I'd longed to hear for more than six weeks. David's voice was scratchy, and his words were garbled and difficult to understand, but I didn't care. Now we could talk. We were finally moving forward.

David was about to enjoy another phase of his new life, something that most of us take for granted: eating. Since David's trach was inserted in the early days of his trauma, his only nourishment was taken through the food drip hanging from an IV pole and feeding into the PEG tube that went directly into his stomach. No appetizing appeal there! Not unless you have a penchant for beige, nondescript, apparently tasteless gloop. Frankly, there was no need for the disgusting-looking liquid to be tasty, since no taste buds would ever be in contact with it.

Once the trach was removed, David underwent a video-fluoroscopy, a test to diagnose the extent of his swallowing difficulties. It showed and recorded his ability to swallow foods, both liquid and solid, and it would determine which foods and drinks were safe for him to ingest.

There are five levels of solid food consistencies, and David eventually would pass through all of them—pureed, minced, ground, chopped, and modified regular foods. His diet first consisted of pureed food—"mushy food," we called it. The fluids had three levels. There were thick fluids, like Jell-O, then there were nectar-thick liquids, like milkshakes, and finally there were thin liquids, such as water and juice.

Meghan, one of David's speech pathologists, and a radiologist, Dave, conducted the test. After they each donned a lead jacket, Dave positioned David in the confines of the fluoroscopy machine and protected him with a lead apron. Dr. Romanno, a rehabilitation specialist, and I watched through a window behind a safe-wall as Meghan spooned barium-coated pudding and bits of cookies between David's lips, and David drank barium-thickened apple juice. Though most of it dripped out, David chewed and swallowed what he was able to trap inside his mouth. We each studied the monitor as the food passed over David's tongue and into his esophagus, taking careful note that the masticated food did not slip into his trachea and into his lungs. Several times I jumped as I saw the food head toward David's windpipe and get caught in a little pocket. Fortunately, his swallow muscles were able to dislodge the food and send it on the right path to his stomach.

When the videofluoroscopy was complete and David was settled into his wheelchair for the ride back to his room, he licked his lips and said, "Mmm, that was good!" He still had traces of the barium stuck to his lips. Meghan, Dave, and I burst into laughter. Meghan said she had never heard anyone describe the barium-laced foods as tasty. David laughed too. I guess when you haven't eaten real food for a while, anything tasted good. This was the first food to touch David's lips in seven weeks. In the coming weeks, videofluoroscopies were administered to David regularly to gauge his eating ability.

Later that day, when David was served his first meal, he devoured it. To him, institutional mashed potatoes and gravy with mashed peas and carrots was a meal fit for a king. He gulped down every last smidgen of food and asked for more. Soon his doctor ordered double portions for him, and like Jack Sprat and his wife in the children's poem, "he licked the platter clean"—breakfast, lunch, and dinner.

Meghan, a speech therapist, began her work with David. She came armed with ice chips and a laryngeal mirror. Because David was afflicted with a swallow disorder, it was Meghan's goal to stimulate his faucial arches, located in the back of the mouth.

Meghan believed that muscle stimulation would trigger David's swallow response so that he'd once again be able to safely swallow foods and drink liquids. Dysphagia, as this disorder is called, stems from the Greek root "dys," which means difficulty, and "phagia," which means to eat.

You've probably never counted your swallows, or even considered them. Swallowing is a natural, automatic process. We swallow hundreds of times each day—foods, liquids, and saliva. A swallow is hardly noticeable, unless a particle of food is aspirated or a liquid gushes down the wrong pipe, causing a coughing reaction. For a person suffering with dysphagia, each swallow is a dangerous chore. Swallowing is the deliberate effort to move food or liquid from the front of the mouth to the rear and then safely into the pharynx, which is the canal that connects to the esophagus. Food must pass into the esophagus and not slip into the air tube, the trachea. The trachea leads to the lungs. If food passes or is aspirated into the lungs, it raises the possibility of pneumonia, which is extremely hazardous.

Getting food into the proper tube is a tricky process. The muscles must simultaneously close off the passageway to the lungs while sending the food into the esophagus. The esophagus, sometimes called the swallow tube, is the final stage before the food enters the stomach. Who would ever think that the seemingly easy process of eating or drinking could be so dangerous? But for those suffering from dysphagia, it is a constant fear. And so with Meghan's help, David would relearn to swallow, to eat, and to drink.

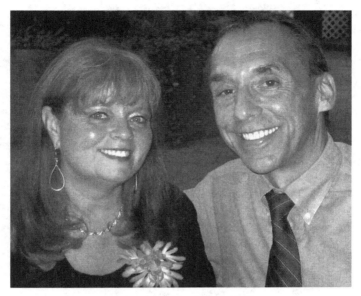

Donna and David, pre TBI

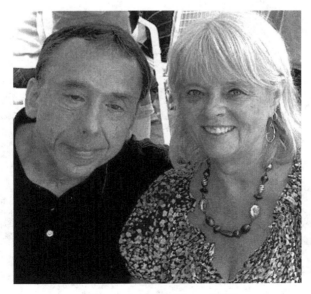

Donna and David, post TBI

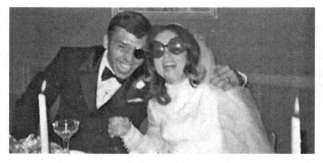

Donna and David on their wedding day (August 9, 1969)

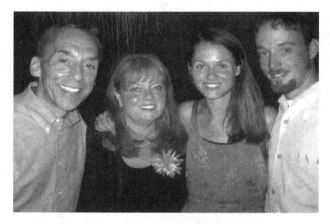

David (pre TBI), Donna, Kiersten, and Jared

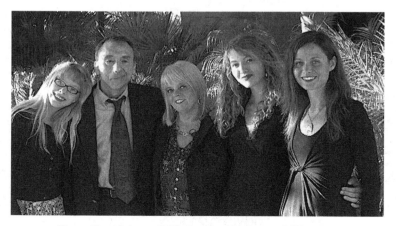

Kaya, David (post TBI), Donna, Treska, and Kiersten

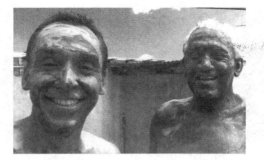

David (pre TBI) and his father, Hank, at a mud bath
near Taos, New Mexico

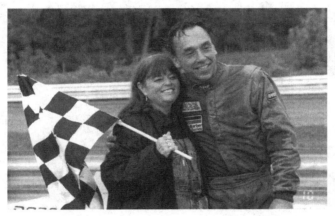

David's first win in the Skip Barber Formula Dodge
race series (November 2000)

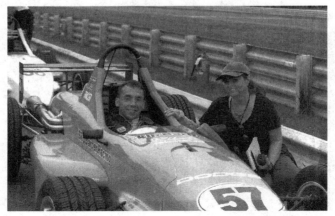

David in a Skip Barber Formula Dodge with Donna

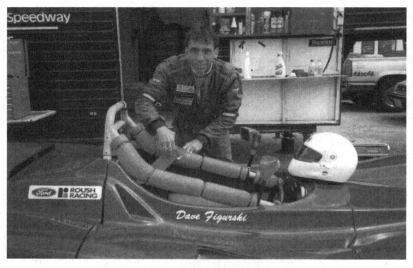

David with a Spec Racer Ford before his SCCA race
at Lime Rock Park

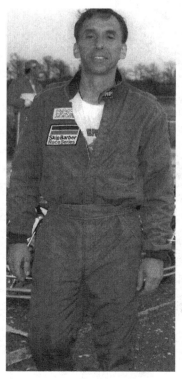

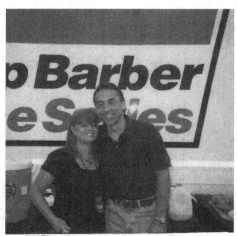

DAVID & DONNA

FIGURSKI

Donna and David at Lime Rock Park

David fully relaxed at the racetrack;
racing was his form of meditation.

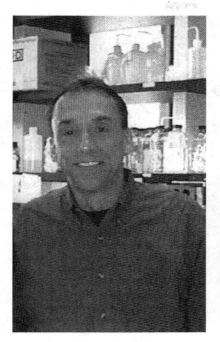

David (pre TBI) in his lab at
Columbia University

David (pre TBI) speaking at Columbia
University

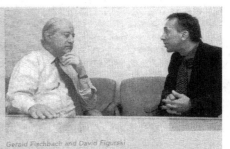

A LONG-AWAITED RETURN David Figurski, Ph.D., professor of
microbiology, who suffered cerebral hemorrhages in January 2005,
returned to CUMC part-time in March. Dr. Figurski received life-sav-
ing surgery at New York–Presbyterian Hospital and has since made
steady progress through rehabilitation therapy with the support of
his wife, children, and grandchildren.

Dr. Figurski has resumed his role as lab head, directing a
research program that focuses on the oral pathogen *Actinobacillus
actinomycetemcomitans*. During his absence, his lab was overseen
by Department of Microbiology colleagues Howard Shuman, Ph.D.,
professor of microbiology; C.S. Hamish Young, Ph.D., professor of
microbiology (retired June'05), and Jonathan Dworkin, Ph.D., assis-
tant professor of microbiology. Dr. Figurski and the Department of Microbiology are particularly grateful to Dr. Dennis Mangan and his
staff at the NIH/NIDCR, who provided invaluable guidance concerning grant management during Dr. Figurski's absence.

Gerald Fischbach and David Figurski

David (post TBI) meeting with the dean of the medical school
on his first day back at work

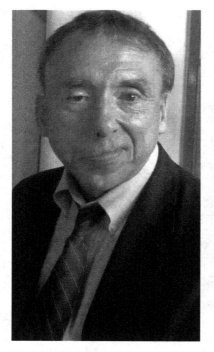

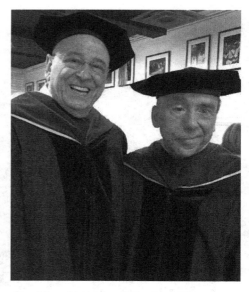

David and his friend, Dr. Saul Silverstein, before David received the Dean's Distinguished Service Award in Basic Science at the medical school graduation in 2017

David at his retirement symposium (August 2013)

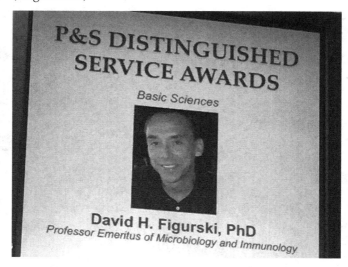

Columbia University's electronic bulletin-board announcing David's award (May 2017); Columbia used a pre TBI photo for the announcement

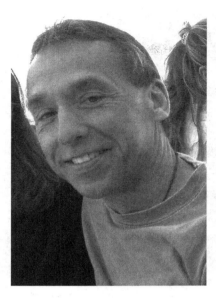

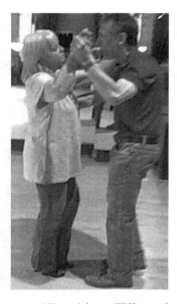

David (pre TBI) summer 2004

Donna and David (post TBI) at a dance lesson with instructor Paula Nieroda

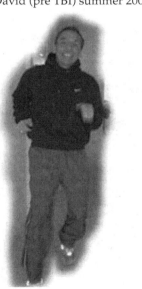

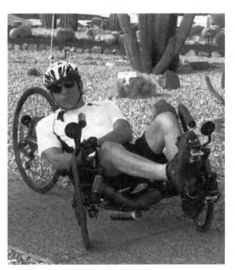

David (pre TBI) models his new winter running clothes for Donna on Christmas Day 2004. This is the last photo of David taken before his TBI. He never ran again

David (post TBI) on his Catrike 700. The recumbent trike gave David his outdoor independence. Between April 2015 and July 2017, David rode 3,579 miles

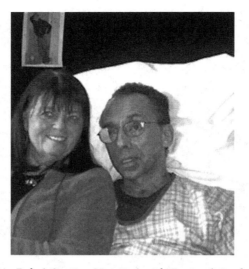

David in Rehabilitation Hospital with Donna (March 2005).
The photo of David on the wall behind his bed was
taken three weeks before his brain injury.

CHAPTER 23

Music for Healing

David's having a roommate brought its own distractions. Avi and his parents had a great support system. Of course, that meant endless visitors. Avi's visitors were loud, but they didn't bother me—at least not in the beginning. I found Avi's visitors to be a welcome diversion. It was early in David's recovery, so he was virtually unaware of their comings and goings. They didn't bother him either.

Many of Avi's visitors acknowledged me when they arrived, but then they quickly forgot about me. I think they also forgot that they were in a hospital room and not at Avi's home. So, though I wasn't included in their conversations, it was impossible not to overhear them.

One day Avi's father, Simon, stopped me in the hallway to tell me that Avi would have many visitors that evening. He said that Avi was a musician and so were his friends, and they wanted to play music for him. Simon asked if David would mind. I knew music was good stimulation for brain-injured patients— that is, if it weren't annoying like the music in the ambulances. Hoping to stimulate David's brain, I'd played music for him on a CD player in the NICU at Columbia-Presbyterian. I told Simon it was fine. I expected a CD player or perhaps an MP3 player. I looked forward to the diversion as another way to pass the time.

About 7:00 p.m., several men lingered in the hallway outside our door. They were dressed from head to toe in black—black trousers, long black jackets over white shirts, and black hats. Many had long beards, though the men were young. They also had earlocks. The men—seven in all—seemed to be waiting, and then they entered the room. Two carried a large keyboard, which they expertly set up. The rest of the men circled Avi's bed. They began to sway and sing or chant. They had beautiful voices. I didn't know the songs, but they were obviously in Hebrew. Some were melodic and calming. Some were rousing and encouraged you to clap your hands.

David seemed to enjoy the music. He showed his enthusiasm by clapping vigorously after each song. Because of his lack of coordination between his right and left side, his clapping was awkward. But that didn't faze him. He clapped anyway. He was enjoying himself for the first time in weeks.

As the weeks moved on, I settled into a routine at Radburn that was dictated by David's schedule. He spent much of his day in therapy—physical, occupational, and speech. Then three meals a day took up much of his time . . . and mine.

Mealtime was a messy adventure. David had to relearn to use a fork and spoon. Forget the knife—too challenging. (It still is.) In the early stages, David didn't need a knife anyway. His food was pureed. It looked like mush. Scrambled eggs, pancakes, applesauce, Jell-O, and puddings were his standard fare.

I arrived early each morning to feed David or to help guide

his hand to his mouth as he relearned to eat. One morning as David was awkwardly spooning scrambled eggs into his mouth with his non-dominant left hand, John, a tall, lanky African-American suffering his own variation of brain trauma, addressed David in a very scratchy, almost unintelligible voice, "Man, put the food in your mouth! It's all down your chin." Not only had soup dribbled down David's chin and the front of his bib, but also the arms of his wheelchair and the floor. Not much made it into David's mouth in those early days as he attempted to feed himself. Like an eighteen-month-old toddler, he wore more food than ever reached his mouth. The sad part was David's obliviousness to the mess he was making. That unawareness also meant he was not embarrassed, as he surely would have been under normal circumstances.

After each meal, David raved, "That was good!" By the end of David's stay at Radburn, almost eight weeks, he was less enamored with the food. He was bored with the mashed potatoes and sometimes declared the meat to be "mystery meat." To mix it up, I began to prepare foods for him from home each day—just for dinner though. He still enjoyed the breakfast foods of scrambled eggs, waffles, and pancakes. He loved his pancakes—still does! Desserts at Radburn always remained in his good graces. He especially liked the desserts of barium-free pudding and Jell-O. He loved the cakes. Each night as the dinner tray was pushed into his room, he'd declare, "Dessert first!" This refrain remained with him for the remainder of his Radburn stay, and I honored it. Dessert first it was.

When David returned home, he still wanted dessert first, but as his food preparer, I refused. He had lost too much weight— nearly thirty pounds. I prepared nutritional meals for him, and I encouraged him to eat them before dessert. I wanted to put some meat on his skeletal frame. His behavior reminded me of my children thirty years ago. They too had to eat dinner before dessert. It felt like history was repeating itself.

David did eat his dinner before dessert. No matter how much or how little dinner he ate, I always gave him dessert—usually a soft cake or a mushy pie. There was little else he enjoyed in his life; I'd see to it he would have dessert. It made me smile to watch his enjoyment.

David's difficulty with eating continues to be a challenge, with possible aspiration always on our minds. David has graduated from the mushy pureed food, though he still enjoys puddings and applesauce. For years he ate applesauce each night as he took his medications. It was kind of like the refrain "A spoonful of sugar makes the medicine go down" I had hummed to my children from Mary Poppins.

Peanut butter and jelly sandwiches have been David's favorite food for lunch. He says they're easy to eat. Pasta and a light tomato sauce, pierogis with cottage cheese and applesauce, and bean burritos and cheese are some of his choice dinners. He tries to eat meats, like pork or chicken, if they are tender and cut into small pieces or shredded. But even so, as his face remains partially paralyzed, they are difficult to chew and make eating a time-consuming chore. There is hope that his swallow will continue to improve. He has made many gains since those early days in the Radburn dining room—no more bibs and no more food dribbling down his chin. John would be proud of him.

Recently, David complained of biting the inside of his mouth. However annoying and uncomfortable that may be, it can only mean that some sensation is returning. He was undoubtedly biting it all along, but now he is feeling it. If his facial paralysis eventually disappears, his swallow muscles will become strong again, and eating will no longer be a dangerous activity. One can only hope.

I enjoyed it whenever friends came. Their visits broke up the tedium and helped to blur the reason why we were in the hospital. It wasn't the way we'd planned to get together, but get together we did . . . at David's bedside. It was interesting to hear some of his friends "speak science" with him—another language entirely. I continued to see David in a new light. I've always been in awe of my husband. He is kind and gentle. His mind is brilliant. His knowledge of molecular biology is vast. I knew he was a well-regarded member of his faculty, but I didn't realize how loved he was by his colleagues until the visits began. His colleagues' sincere fondness for him was apparent. I burst with pride.

Saul made the trip across the Hudson River to Radburn to visit David numerous times. As chairman of the department, no doubt he was checking on David to be sure he was not playing hooky from work. "When are you getting out of that bed? You have a lab to run," he would say in mock seriousness. I liked it when Saul visited. I knew I'd laugh. I needed that.

Aaron (Dr. Aaron Mitchell) also visited. Though we'd met on numerous occasions at Columbia functions, I didn't really know Aaron. But during the next months, I got to know him well. He visited every weekend—sometimes both Saturday and Sunday. He spent hours with David, updating him about the happenings at the lab, discussing science techniques and principles, and reassuring David that his students were hard at work and their projects were progressing.

One Saturday morning in March, David and Aaron sat in the lounge. David, in his wheelchair and barely cognizant of his world, looked at Aaron and most seriously said that he (meaning himself) needed to begin preparations for the departmental retreat, which occurred each September. David was the retreat organizer. I didn't know whether to laugh or cry. The retreat was six months away, and David's sense of responsibility was shining through. That was a good sign.

But I was alarmed too. I was frightened that David did not realize that he was unable to organize the retreat this year. He could barely move from his bed to his wheelchair—and even then he needed assistance. I couldn't understand why he didn't comprehend this. What had happened to his brain? I met Aaron's eyes with apprehension, but I was soon relieved when Aaron, without missing a beat, assured David that the retreat preparations were underway and that he needn't worry. Aaron insisted then that David be well enough to attend. I smiled when David promised that he wouldn't miss it.

My cousins dropped by too. They always brought good cheer and distraction. David's students and postdocs came, bringing questions about their projects. I also enjoyed when the nursing aides took time from their busy days to chat for a few minutes. So although the days were long, there were pleasant distractions mixed in for both David and me, for which we were grateful.

CHAPTER 24

ETR (Expected Time for Recovery)

Each day had the same routine. David, though awake and taking part in his therapies, responding to his doctors and nurses, and showing definite signs of cognition, was still unaware of the seriousness of his illness. That was probably good. I understood—or at least I thought I did. Truthfully, comprehension of the magnitude of David's trauma was beyond my realization at that point.

I didn't yet realize the patience, persistence, time, and downright hard work that David's brain injury would demand of me. And like David, it was a good thing I was not fully aware. It would have been unbearable. Oh, I wasn't ignorant. I didn't have my head in the sand—not by that time. I knew it was serious, more serious than anything I had ever experienced in my entire life. I knew it would impact our lives. I just didn't know yet how drastically.

Dr. Connolly, the neurosurgeon who performed two of three of David's brain surgeries, said that David would probably be in rehabilitation for nearly six months. That meant David and I would have to live apart—a forever amount of time it seemed. Though I hated it, I had to keep a positive spin on it. I had to believe David would get better and that our lives would return to normal. And I had to live in the moment. If we had to live apart for David to recover, so be it. I couldn't change that. The past was obviously gone, and life as we knew it would never again be the same. I couldn't think about the future. It was simply too scary. I didn't know what it would present, but then nobody ever really does. I never told David about the anticipated length of his recovery. I didn't think he'd handle it well, and frankly, he wasn't aware enough anyway in his early weeks at Radburn to comprehend its implications. I don't know what he thought he was in the hospital for, but I was certain he expected to be released within days—not weeks or months. I wouldn't deflate his hopes.

Later, after David had been released from Radburn, we met with Dr. Connolly at Columbia-Presbyterian Hospital for a follow-up check. Dr. Connolly explained that, although he was unable to predict how long a recovery period to expect, it would take David years to regain his physical abilities, maybe five or more years. *Wow! Who has five years to lose?* I thought. But we had no choice. Healing from a traumatic brain injury takes time . . . lots of time. Many people do not survive the extensive damage that a brain injury inflicts. I had *no* idea how much time, and to think I freaked out over five years—can you imagine how I feel over more than twelve years later? That's how far past the event we are now. It seems so inconceivable, yet true!

Many suffer with cognitive deficits that affect thinking, memory, or reasoning skills. In that, David was lucky. The cognitive part of his brain was intact. Sensory processing is in another area. In that part of the brain, the five senses of sight, taste, smell, touch, and hearing may be altered. David's vision was severely damaged, and his sense of taste was altered. That may have been why he preferred dessert when he had rarely eaten dessert previously. Those taste buds worked best.

He could taste sweetness. The rest of his senses seemed to be working properly.

The communication area of the brain, which involves both expression and understanding, is another part of the brain that can become severely damaged. This area was affected, but David is now able to communicate and process speech relatively normally. Though his speech is slower than it was pre-trauma and he hasn't regained his quality of voice, as time passes, he's become more and more intelligible. He has even been an invited speaker at conferences in his field of molecular biology.

A brain trauma can also affect both the mental and the behavioral health of a patient. This can result in depression, anxiety, aggression, or personality disorders. Fortunately, the trauma did not affect David's mental or behavioral health. He was affected, however, in many other areas. While David was still in a coma, it was difficult to know what challenges he would have to deal with. His doctors could make predictions due to their observations, but, until David was actually able to do things, it was not certain what he would be dealing with.

In the early months, David suffered from bladder dysfunction. Though this problem has lessened, David still has major concerns and needs to know where the nearest restroom is in any situation. He still fights the battle against an ataxic right hand and arm, which seem to have minds of their own. His balance remains severely impaired, though slowly progresses, and his swallow disorder continues to make eating and drinking fluids a challenge. I think that, though each and every one of the deficits is a horror in itself, for me the hardest to bear would have been a loss of either his cognitive brain or a personality change—a change from the fairly calm, gentle man I married to an aggressive, disturbed person I would no longer recognize.

Though we are not happy about any of David's disabilities and we wish this nightmare had never befallen us, we remind each other often: "It beats the alternative!" David is alive.

So each day, I set off to the hospital with a smile on my lips and hope in my heart. My goal was to bolster David's spirits and to keep my hope alive.

CHAPTER 25

Close Living Wears Thin

Our visitors added another dimension to our routine and gave us hope, but it was Avi, his family, and his visitors who really added color. I was glad for the companionship of Avi's parents, Rebekah and Simon. I appreciated our conversations centered on either Avi or David. After all, they were the people we were concerned about most. It was easy living with Avi and his parents. Simon, Rebekah, Avi, David, and I lived and breathed together hour after hour in a small two-bed room.

Rebekah and Simon observed Shabbat every week. The Sabbath begins on Friday evening at dusk, as the sun lowers in the sky. It ends one hour after sunset on Saturday. Oh, the flurry each Friday afternoon as Rebekah and Simon prepared for their weekly holy day. Bags of groceries crowded the room, a microwave oven sat ready on a table, and a crockpot was set to cooking their Saturday dinner for when Shabbat ended. They devoted much of Friday night and Saturday to prayer. No visitors were allowed. It was a quiet, calm, and peaceful time.

Sundays, though, were the antithesis of Saturdays. They seemed like party days. Nonstop visitors streamed in, setting the pattern for the rest of the week—until Shabbat arrived again. At first, the endless visitors didn't bother anyone, least of all David or Avi. They were on another plane. But as weeks passed, David's awareness heightened, and the close living began to wear thin. Avi's visitors became a strain. David grew agitated by the constant din. The number of people was overwhelming. Upwards of five visitors for Avi, exceeding the hospital's regulations, often crowded into the room.

David's discomfort set me on edge too. The loud voices of Avi's friends and relatives and his visitors' disregard for David's comfort annoyed me. I could not then, nor do I yet, understand their insensitivity. It baffles me still that they used inappropriate outside voices in a hospital room with brain-injured patients, who often react adversely to loud stimuli. Didn't they realize that raising their voices would not make Avi more aware? It reminded me of how people often raise their voices while speaking to foreigners, thinking it will make them understand. It doesn't work. Avi too was unable to respond just because they yelled their greetings.

Perhaps I was partially to blame. I had never objected to their booming voices before, so I suppose they thought it was acceptable. But in the beginning their loud chatter hadn't troubled David, so it didn't bother me either. I felt that if Avi's visitors were helpful to him and they didn't impede David's recovery, then it was okay. All that changed in the middle of March.

Possibly it was the strain of my being confined to hospitals for more than two months. Perhaps it was the tension of the close living. The walls of the tiny room seemed to be closing in on me. Maybe it was the smell of boiled cabbage and other strange odors emanating from the crockpot clinging to the walls and lingering in the air for days. It may have been directly related to David's heightened awareness. But I think mostly it was the lack of respect by some of Avi's visitors that sent me toppling over the edge.

One day, David seemed especially disturbed by two of Avi's visitors. David had been suffering from a urinary tract infection for the past week. It broke my heart to see him in pain, and I was helpless to do anything, causing me more stress. The few moments that David could sleep were a welcome respite for both him and me. But David's sleep was not on the agenda with Avi's loud visitors.

An elderly gentleman, one of Avi's visitors, entered the room and settled in near the far wall of the room. He attempted a yelling conversation. Avi was oblivious, but David was not. David began showing serious signs of agitation. When I could no longer pacify David, I asked Rebekah to remind her visitors to use quiet voices. She seemed apologetic and readily agreed. Nevertheless, after a few minutes, the elderly man continued to speak in a booming voice. David's agitation grew, and I repeated my request to Rebekah. This time I also addressed her visitor. I suggested that Avi might hear him more easily if he moved closer to the head of Avi's bed. He moved a few inches closer to the foot of the bed, but his volume remained the same. I was relieved when he soon left.

My relief was short-lived, as a new set of guests arrived. A young woman and man took the elderly man's place. They too came with jubilant voices. The scenario was repeated, and David's agitation heightened. After waiting a few moments, hoping that Rebekah would quiet her guests, I poked my head around the curtain and once more made my request for quieter voices. Rebekah agreed to intervene, but if she did, nothing changed. I tried to soothe David, but he was beyond calming. I worried that his blood pressure would rise. I feared further damage to his brain. He was seriously distressed. As I rounded the curtain for the third time to make one last plea, David grabbed the curtain between his and Avi's beds. In his nearly unintelligible, guttural, gravelly voice, he "yelled" at Avi to tell his guests to be quiet. Of course, Avi could do nothing. Rebekah stood mute—shocked by David's unexpected outburst. The young woman stared at David . . . then raucously laughed at him!

I was stunned by her insensitive and inhumane behavior. I stared into her eyes and said, "This is a brain injury ward. I am sorry that you think this is funny!" I made a final attempt to calm David. Then I walked directly to the nurse's station.

The nurses expected me. They probably even waged bets on when I would finally break—not particularly for this event, but for a long list of infractions since the beginning of February: the loud visitors, the weekly crockpot cooking, the stacks of boxes with their unknown contents lining the walls and overflowing into the bathroom, the chanting and keyboard sessions, the constant ring of cell phones and the accompanying chatter of phone conversations, and the men who rudely refused to retract their legs sprawled across the passageway, forcing me to crawl over them. Since Avi's arrival, the nurses and doctors asked if they should intervene. I refused. I have a lot of patience, and as long as it didn't bother David, I didn't mind. But the rude man and the laughing girl were the straws that made me break.

The nurses nodded knowingly. They seemed relieved to finally be able to intervene and prevent some of the nonsense. They knew it was a matter of time before I broke . . . and I did. I later spoke to the doctor in charge, and he assured me there would be a change. The next day David was moved to a private room just outside the lockdown unit.

The change to the private room was a relief—not only for David, but also for me. The simpler life probably lowered my blood pressure. I should have requested it earlier, but a change of room or roommate could have been disastrous. I knew what we were up against with Avi. I did not know what issues an unknown new roommate would bring. I feared a roommate like the man down the hall who, day and night, bellowed and cursed incessantly at the nurses and aides and at nobody at all. I'll leave the phrases to your imagination. To include them in this book would rate it X. Or David could have been relocated near the room of the fifty-something-year-old woman who moaned, "Mooommmyyy, Mooommmyyy, Mooommmyyy" her every waking moment. Her woeful cry traveled the distance of the hallway. Like the man's curses, her cries were relentless.

These patients were locked within their own form of brain damage, and though I was sympathetic to their suffering, I knew that subjecting David to the clamor would not be beneficial to his mental health. It wouldn't have been good for mine either. The fear of rooming near either of them kept me from complaining about Avi's family and friends. But the young woman's laughing at David in his brain-injured state was the catalyst for the next part of our adventure at Radburn.

I entered our new "home" armed with a tape dispenser. I taped photos of David—pre-trauma—on every inch of exposed wall: David in his jogging suit and in his racecar, pictures of David with his arms draped around his granddaughters, David and me laughing, pictures to remind him of who he was, and pictures of memories to bring him back to me. I had an ulterior motive too. I wanted his doctors, nurses, and aides to see who David was before the assault on his brain transformed him into a bed-ridden body with no personality and no sense of being.

Next I placed the get-well plants and cards from family and friends on the windowsill. I made that room ours, comfortable and cozy. I pushed out thoughts of who slept in that bed before David and what miseries these walls held. It was our room, and I was grateful.

CHAPTER 26

Prisoners without Bars

I was pleased and surprised when, one night as I glanced through the window of the lockdown door, I saw a familiar face. It was Judy Thau. Her face was drawn and etched with stress. She looked more drained than when I had seen her last.

Judy and I met during the last week of David's stay at Columbia-Presbyterian. I noticed her in the waiting room, around her hearth, surrounded by family. Yes, we both broke the rules of the Clan according to Jean Auel. Our meeting was inevitable. We were drawn to each other. We stole glances until finally our eyes locked. I saw her pain. She saw mine. Hers was fresh. Mine seemed age-old, although it had been only nineteen days. I wanted to help, but we didn't talk, not right away. One day as she sat alone, I approached hesitantly. Eventually we talked, and our stories poured out.

Judy's husband, Steve, suffered a traumatic brain injury on January 31st, only weeks after David. Steve was tethered to a set of machines in a NICU room at Columbia-Presbyterian. He was just a few cubicles from David. Though Judy and I each had our own support systems and were surrounded by family and friends, we recognized the desperation in each other's eyes. I wanted to ease her pain. Judy and I became instant friends. As a veteran of my own nightmare for nearly three weeks, I hoped to offer beneficial information about the process. Our parallel fears of losing our husbands, who were our best friends, bound us together. So when I saw Judy's beautiful face through the window of the lockdown unit at Radburn, I was excited. Relief flooded me too. Though family and friends held my hand and offered support and love, it was Judy who truly understood what I was feeling because she was feeling it too.

We talked. We compared stories of our husbands' traumas. We remembered our lives before trauma, though those lives seemed to be lost. We learned that our life-stories were similar. Only a few years separate Judy and me, I being the elder. I met David when I was sixteen years old and knew in an instant that we would someday marry. And we did when I turned twenty. Judy also knew at an early age that she would marry Steve. She was only twelve when they met. We'd been with these men for many, many years, and our commitment to them ran deep. Coincidentally, David and Steve share the same numbers for their trauma days. David owns 13, while Steve's day is 31—both in the month of January.

When the therapists realized that Judy and I were friends, they conveniently arranged for David's and Steve's therapy schedules to coincide. This allowed Judy and me to occasionally meet for coffee and a chat—that is, to lean on each other. Most of the time, though, Judy ran errands or entertained family, while I leaned against the wall in the gym, silently encouraging David.

Through the years, Judy and I have remained good friends. Though we live too far to visit often, we have been to each other's home, and we have met in New York City for an occasional lunch and a catch-up chat. Of course, phone and email keep us tethered to each other's life. I am immensely grateful for Judy's friendship, her understanding, and her laughter.

Though family and friends are well-meaning, offer encouragement, and often remind David and me how fortunate we are, they simply cannot comprehend how our lives were ripped apart. They cannot know how our dreams of travel and racing, how Friday and Saturday night movies and dinners, and how weekend walks in the park have been stripped from our lives. Yes, even something as simple as a walk in the park has vanished. Judy understands. Her life is in tatters too. I know I'm lucky. I'm fortunate to have my husband and best friend with me still. But to hear even the most well-meaning friends, whose lives are intact, tell me I am lucky can be hard to bear.

I don't blame them for not understanding. How can they? It hasn't affected their lives. Those unfortunate enough to suffer through TBI with a loved one, a mother or father, son or daughter, find the consequences to be almost unbearable, and they definitely are. But to live through TBI with your spouse and very best friend affects your every waking moment and your sleeping ones too. It changes your life like you cannot imagine. Most family and friends, after lending their much-needed support, return to their own lives. It's normal. It's natural. But with TBI, the crisis does not end for the patient or the spouse. Months and years may pass before life can, if you are "lucky," resume a degree of normalcy. For David and me, life, even after more than twelve years, is still not normal. It may be selfish of me, but I want our old life back. Who wouldn't?

But what's worse is being the person saddled with TBI—being David. He's locked inside his body—a prisoner without bars. No one who is not a prisoner of TBI himself can fully grasp the anguish. Not even I, who am closest to David, can fully comprehend his life and his fears. But, I too am a prisoner without bars. I am a prisoner of David's life. I am his constant caregiver. Remember in the early part of this story when I said that David is my best friend and I begged each neurosurgeon to give him back to me—no matter what? I meant it! Caring for David—loving him—is my choice.

So I say, "It is not luck being saddled with TBI." It would've been luck, I think, never to have heard the words "traumatic brain injury" or never to have learned the dire meaning of them. It would have been lucky to have our lives continue on their paths without TBI. I think Judy would agree.

I never regretted the move to the private room. The calmer atmosphere added a measure of peace to our days. David slowly crawled out of the abyss that his mind had plunged him into eight weeks prior.

I prepared PowerPoint presentations of some of my students' poetry on my computer. With the font set at 100, it was possible for David to see the screen and decipher the letters. His vision was blurry, tilted, and double, and his speech remained garbled. With my students' silly poems and some nonsense sentences that I made up, David exercised his eyes and practiced enunciating words. I made him work in that hospital. No lolling around in bed for him!

During rehabilitation therapy, David tottered down the hallway clinging to his walker to reinforce his balance as he learned to walk again. Patients who spend extended time in a hospital often lose muscle tone in their legs. They must be strengthened in order for the patients to become ambulatory again. Unfortunately, this was not the problem with David. The brain injury had affected his balance, and so, although his muscles were strong, his balance was off-kilter. As a result, he was not able to walk unassisted. It would be years before David could walk on his own again, and even after twelve years, he can only walk unassisted indoors.

Each night before David went to bed, I massaged his feet and legs to calm him. I read to him too—books about his racing passion. *Racers* by Richard Williams, the story of F1 drivers Michael Schumacher, Jacques Villeneuve, and Damon Hill, and *Gilles Villenueve*, written by Gerald Donaldson, were just two of the books I read aloud. I learned a lot about David's racing heroes, and it passed the time pleasantly. David was an attentive listener. It was about the only thing he could do well.

Kiersten arrived again from New Mexico with her daughters Treska and Kaya for David's last weeks at Radburn. The private room was a lifesaver for us then. The girls spent hours entertaining their grandfather. They danced. They sang. They crawled on his bed for quiet grandpa talks. The girls did most of the talking. David's voice was weak and scratchy. His speech therapist encouraged him to practice the "eee" sound to strengthen his vocal chords, but as cooperative as David was with all suggestions by his therapists, he completely resisted this request. He ignored my pleas too. He listened only to Treska. With her, he would practice his "eee" sound, and she loved screeeching with her grandfather.

Easter fell on March 27th while Kiersten and the girls were still visiting. I applied for an overnight pass so David could come home. I wanted to make our traditional holiday meal—baked ham with horseradish on the side, sweet and hot sausage, scalloped potatoes, corn, and hot, buttered rolls. David loves that meal, and I knew he would enjoy watching the girls hunt for Easter eggs. The nurses told me the hospital encouraged weekend passes for patients before their actual release to adapt to home life again and to work out any kinks, so I thought this would be perfect. But my request was denied. I was disappointed. So was David.

I was not deterred. If David was unable to come home for dinner, dinner would come to him—even if I had to cook all night. It turned out that I didn't have to cook at all. My cousin Patti prepared our traditional ham dinner and delivered it to Radburn on Easter afternoon. We (Patti and Bryce, Kiersten, Treska and Kaya, and David and I) celebrated in the sixth floor dining room with several other families who apparently had the same idea. The dinner was wonderful. David loved it. It was his first non-institutional food in two-and-a-half months—other than the food I slipped him, of course. That day reminded me of the proverb "If life deals you lemons, make lemonade." We enjoyed a lot of "lemonade" that Easter.

CHAPTER 27

April Fool's Joke?

The insurance company began to worry about David's progress. They didn't believe he was making gains fast enough to warrant remaining under hospital care. That simply was not true! The therapists touted daily David's amazing progress. The simple fact was that the company wanted to cut its losses. Radburn, to its credit, intervened on David's behalf. Their efforts allowed David to receive all but one week of his allotted insurance time. My stress soared each week as David's therapists reported his progress and we waited for the insurance company's decision.

With the realization that David would soon be sent home with a feeding tube protruding from his belly and a urine bag strapped to his leg, I became more proactive. I insisted to the doctor that they wean David from the Foley catheter to a condom catheter before he left the hospital. Dr. Romanno brushed my concern off and assured me that many patients return home with a catheter. I informed him that this patient would not.

Dr. Romanno argued that the visiting nurse could remove the Foley catheter. I was incredulous! Had he forgotten that David had already experienced horrific pain in the hospital on the two occasions nurses attempted to wean him from the Foley catheter? How could Dr. Romanno possibly believe that a visiting nurse could accomplish this feat at home? When I reminded him of these episodes, he simply told me that I could take David to the emergency room if a problem arose. What was he thinking? I questioned his medical expertise. I had no doubt the Foley catheter would have to be reinserted. In the past, David's pain had escalated quickly, and it was only relieved by reinserting the catheter. What good would going to an emergency room accomplish? That was not a solution. David needed twenty-four-hour supervision to accomplish the weaning process. For two weeks, I suggested that Dr. Romanno make an appointment with the urologist. For two weeks, he did nothing.

Then Saul, my magic man, visited. I invited Dr. Romanno into David's room and made polite introductions. "Dr. Silverstein meet Dr. Romanno; Dr. Romanno meet Dr. Silverstein." But there was nothing polite after that. Saul told Dr. Romanno very frankly that he was not doing his job. He told him he needed David back in his lab. Dr. Romanno attempted his brush-it-under-the-rug tactic with Saul, the same tactic he repeatedly used with me. When his evasive tactic didn't work with Saul, Dr. Romanno raised his voice to talk over Saul, another strategy Dr. Romanno had used repeatedly with me. This technique also was ineffective with Saul. Dr. Romanno was no match for Dr. Silverstein.

I got into the fray too. I told Dr. Romanno that he needed to listen to his patients. His visits with a smile on his face were useless. Though he asked probing questions ("Are you in pain?"), he didn't listen to the answers. He heard, but he didn't listen. Dr. Romanno again tried to be evasive with Saul and me, but he was not successful. We would not let him leave the room without listening to us. A lot of banter flew over David's bed. Finally Saul instructed Dr. Romanno to make an appointment with the urologist. Within minutes the appointment was made.

Thank you, Saul!

Since the urologist, located at Maplecreek Center in New Jersey, did not make calls at Radburn, it fell on me to drive David to him. In retrospect, I wondered why an ambulance wasn't ordered for transport or why I was permitted, even encouraged, to drive David myself. How safe was that? But at the time, I was relieved that we finally had an appointment, and I didn't question the decision. It was March and very cold outside. I bundled David up, settled him into my SUV with the help of an aide, and we set off in search of Maplecreek. Another adventure! I felt as if we were playing hooky from the hospital. The trip had an air of excitement.

I liked the urologist. He was thorough, and David was finally being treated. The urologist performed a complete urological workup on David. The result was that there was nothing seriously wrong. He said it would take time for David's normal bladder function to return. Unfortunately, the doctor was not able to predict when that might be.

When we returned to Radburn, the Foley catheter was again removed. There was anxiety, of course, but this time David was closely watched and the condom catheter was finally successful.

While the condom catheter meant we were getting close to normal, life was so far from normal it was almost comical. But not really. The insurance company determined David's release date would be Friday, April 1st. Was this someone's bizarre humor—an April Fool's joke? David was not well enough to come home. He was totally dependent on the nursing and aide staff. But he *was* coming home. Without ever setting eyes on David, his insurance company determined his wellness and the state of his health. The insurance company refused to pay for any more care. I have only one word—ludicrous!

During the days before his release, David's therapists

trained me to move him safely from bed to wheelchair and wheelchair to toilet. The nursing staff demonstrated how to feed him and pour water through the PEG tube that led directly into his stomach. They showed me how to hygienically change the dressing while allowing no germs to enter his body. I was instructed in which medications to give David, how many, and the time of day he needed to take each. No easy task! He took about fifteen different pills. The nurses demonstrated how to put drops and ointment into his eyes and told me to patch his right eye every night. I was overwhelmed. It was Nursing 101, 102, and 103 all rolled into a few short days.

I am a teacher. I teach children to read and write. I am an expert on teaching addition, subtraction, multiplication, and division. I can choreograph the learning activities of twenty-five or more children, and I can even wrap Band-Aids on non-existent boo-boos. But I am not a nurse. Yet that is what I had to become—without the degree and without the pay. I did not know how I could handle this by myself. I was excited and looking forward to David's return home. But I dreaded it too, so I was grateful that Kiersten was there to offer some transitional assistance.

April 1st came, and David said goodbye to the nursing staff, the aides, and to his therapists. I took pictures of the dear people who played a pivotal role in our lives. Most he'll never remember, but I will never forget. I hoped the pictures would jog David's memory to allow him to know the caregivers who encouraged him to get better.

Finally I strapped David into my SUV for the trek home. It felt good, but it was strange too. We were greeted with balloons blowing in the breeze from our stoop. A "Welcome Home" sign was draped over the garage door. My cousin Patti was spreading her good cheer again. This would be the start of a new adventure—one for which David and I were not ready.

CHAPTER 28

Barely Staying Sane

Kiersten and her daughters proved to be wonderful distractions as David and I transitioned from Radburn to home, but soon they returned to their home in New Mexico. Next, my brother John arrived from Phoenix with his fresh expertise on how to care for a brain-injured patient. He was still caring for his son, who suffered a TBI only three months earlier. But in the four days alone with David between Kiersten's departure and John's arrival, I nearly lost my mind.

David went through a lot of stages on his journey to recovery. Like an infant, he relied on me for his every need. If you've had children, you probably remember the terrible twos—maybe not so fondly. Two-year-olds are self-centered. They think the world revolves around them. David went through that stage. It was all me, me, me. He needed constant attention. About that time, I started to get sick of my name. "Donna, can you get me some ____?" "Donna, where is my ____?" "Donna, I need ____." (Slot anything into those empty spaces.) Fortunately, the terrible two stage ends. It was followed by the "sweet years," when the child loves his or her parents to bits. David made up for his terrible two stage during this phase. The next stage David traveled through was the teen years. He was a combination of delightful and disagreeable, but we got through it. When he finally reached the adult years, I was grateful that each of these stages passed quickly—almost as though they were fast-forwarded. I'd already raised two children; I wasn't expecting this big kid.

David's need for constant care left me sleep-deprived and without a waking moment of peace. If I wasn't setting out David's pills, cleaning his PEG dressing, preparing mushy food for him, making smoothies in the blender, or rushing him to the bathroom, I was doing laundry, paying bills, and generally cleaning up in his wake. How could one person be so needy? The chores were endless. I felt captive in my own home. I could not leave for even a moment—not to walk down the street to get the mail, and certainly not to run to the grocery store less than a mile away.

I was frightened even to leave David's side for fear of an accident. His needs were great. He was totally disabled, so I was his arms and his legs. David was like a car whose engine had stalled. He could do nothing for himself. Fortunately, our main living area has the kitchen, living room, dining room, and my office within steps of each other. Only when David napped on the couch was I able to log onto my computer to make contact with the outside world yet still keep a vigilant watch.

Nighttime seemed to be more harrowing than the waking hours. I welcomed the darkness with the hope of getting rest, but resting never happened. I set up a bedroom for us in my office, so David would not have to tackle the stairs to our third-floor bedroom. Another bathroom was within a few steps. This seemed to be the most practical solution. We slept on a pullout couch. I placed his pillows at a forty-five-degree angle, but even in this nearly upright position, David's swallow disorder made him sit up every few minutes to cough. It sounded as though he were choking to death. This did not allow peaceful sleep for him or for me.

Also, David felt a need to urinate every two hours. Though the condom catheter was in place, he was unable to understand that he did not physically need to use the bathroom. So, whenever he felt the urge to urinate, he tried to crawl out of bed. Since he was not able to stand, I feared he would fall and break an arm or a leg. So, I slept—if that's what it was—with one eye open. It seemed that every few moments I needed to jump out of bed and rush to restrain David.

I then made a barricade of sofa cushions and stacked them against David's side of the bed. I hoped the barrier would deter him enough to allow me to dash around the bed to get him into his wheelchair safely. That system worked a few times, but one night, he refused to wait. By the time I reached him, he had broken through the barrier, threw the cushions aside, pushed his wheelchair away, and in his wild panic to get to the bathroom threw me against the bookcase. I was stunned. His behavior frightened me. I'd never seen David act in a violent manner. It took what seemed like hours for me to settle him.

I longed for my brother to arrive—for the relief I felt he would bring. I was terrified—scared of my own husband. As I expected, John arrived with a sense of calmness. He was little more than two weeks ahead of me in the TBI process. He was my forerunner. Understanding the needs of his son helped him to know what I might need to assist David.

John brought an extra suitcase filled with tools. He transformed my house into a safe haven for David. John attached safety grab-bars in the bathroom and in doorways. He hung shelving in the laundry room to accommodate David's extra equipment. He worked with David, his friend, and kept him company. John's presence gave me the freedom to shop for the food and supplies that I would need for the weeks to come. Soon John returned home. I was sad to see my brother leave, but grateful for his help and support.

I was grateful too for my son, who arrived a few days later to stay for a week. He helped arrange and schedule the medical assistants who would be attending to David's needs for the next few weeks. It was difficult to juggle the schedules for David's physical, occupational, and speech therapists, as well as his nurse and a nurse's aide. We had to accommodate their schedules, yet not overlap their visits. David needed resting time too. Our home was invaded by strangers for several weeks—people arriving and departing all day long.

The nurse aide's schedule was the easiest. She came each morning at about eight o'clock and stayed until eleven o'clock. She got David up from bed and showered and shaved him before getting him dressed. She made breakfast for him and did a variety of household chores, like vacuuming, emptying the dishwasher, and making the bed. She was delightful, and I wished I could have kept her services indefinitely, but her help ended when I decided that home therapy was not best for David. I believed he needed more aggressive therapy than what was being offered in our home. I arranged for outpatient therapy at Radburn, the same facility where David had been an inpatient.

Soon Jared had to leave too. It seemed like I was saying a lot of goodbyes. But before Jared left, Betty arrived.

CHAPTER 29

Betty

Betty stayed with us for almost three months. She is a friend of my daughter. Kiersten studied a summer in Germany while pursuing her degree in German Women's History at Bard College. When she graduated, she wanted nothing more than to live in Germany, and so, upon her graduation, she moved to Regensburg. It was in Regensburg, in the heart of Bavaria, that she met Falko, her husband-to-be. Soon they left that beautiful, ancient city on the Danube River and moved to Falko's hometown of Leipzig, where both of their daughters were born. While Kiersten lived in Leipzig, she met sixteen-year-old Betty, who lived with her parents, sister, and brothers in Kiersten's apartment building. Kiersten and Betty became friends, and Betty babysat Kiersten's oldest daughter, Treska. It was this friendship that brought Betty to us four years later.

Kiersten contacted Betty in March to ask her if she would be interested in living with David and me when David was released from the hospital. She enticed Betty by offering her her own bedroom and bathroom and convinced her that it would be a wonderful opportunity to experience life in America. I had reservations and was certain that David would object. We enjoyed our privacy. Kiersten assured me that I'd love Betty, and David was too sick to protest. Since I was overwhelmed and needed help with David, I set my reservations aside.

Though Betty had visited Kiersten in Taos, she'd never been to New York. She was excited, and I was glad for her company. Betty stayed with David during the day, allowing me to return to my classroom to teach my first graders. In the evenings, Betty often helped prepare dinner with me, and we chatted. But it was after dinner that David, Betty, and I spent hours together around the table talking and laughing, drawing closer and closer—becoming a new family. David had a very lively sense of humor at that time, and we laughed a lot. About 9:00 p.m., after I put David to bed, I'd work on my computer and Betty would work on the one that we loaned her . . . when she wasn't practicing the guitar.

Betty is an accomplished cellist, but, unfortunately, she didn't bring her cello with her. She thought it would disturb us. She was wrong. We would've loved it. So, I did the next best thing. I loaned her my guitar. Though Betty had never played the guitar, she diligently practiced each evening and was soon strumming the chords and picking the strings like a pro. Strains of classical music drifted on the night air. It was calming—what I needed. I insisted that she bring her cello the next time she visited. She promised. That girl makes beautiful music.

After some weeks passed, I asked Betty why she came. She didn't know us, and she was far from home. She said she liked Kiersten and was sure she'd like her parents too. She added that she also wanted to know New York City and felt this was a good opportunity. It was perfect—for all of us.

Betty often hopped on the bus at the bottom of the hill to commute the thirty- to sixty-minute trip to the City. She was methodical about her exploration of New York. During the week, while David spent hours answering email, Betty searched the web, planning which neighborhood to explore next. She saw and experienced more of New York in the few months she lived with us than I did in the many years I lived at its edge.

In an email to me years after her visit, Betty still had clear memories of her time touring the City. She visited the Metropolitan Museum of Art twice, enjoyed a film of the history of the City in the Museum of the City of New York, and saw her first jellyfish at the aquarium. In Central Park, she saw a Shakespeare play and enjoyed watching people play the strange, to her, sport of baseball, which "doesn't really exist in Europe."

A few weeks after Betty arrived, I asked David if he'd like to trek to Erie, to visit his father. Hank hadn't seen David since David's initial hospitalization. Of course, David had been in a coma then and was unaware of his father's presence. I thought the visit would be good for both of them.

What was I thinking? I must have had a brain lapse! David was like a limp rag. He could not move on his own. I had to physically move him from bed or chair to wheelchair. A long car trip would certainly be a challenge for both of us. But once I made the offer, I couldn't rescind it. It would've been cruel. Surprisingly, David jumped at the idea of going to Erie. And so did Betty. At least I thought she did.

Later Betty confessed that the trip frightened her. She said it posed additional uncertainty in this strange, new land. The added ambiguity was scary. She wrote:

To me that meant more new things and therefore, insecurity. But I quickly saw that it actually was a good idea to go there and everything else worked fine, so I never again had doubts about having come . . . I think we spent the whole time together and that was good for getting used to each other. I think there always was this, how can I say that, atmosphere or spirit of enjoying life and enjoying the day and the rest

doesn't matter. Making the best out of everything . . . I felt like being
part of your family and that was great. I had the impression that what
I did was appreciated and useful.

The trip worried me too, but my anxiety was different from
Betty's angst. I was concerned I was in over my head. The drive
was long—more than ten hours. I was supposed to be in charge,
but what if I got on the road, far from the security of home, and I
couldn't handle David? That terrified me. I admit I was excited
too. For months, the hospitals held David captive, and now it
seemed that his home was his prison. I hoped that a change
of scene would defy his illness. My excitement conquered my
concerns. Setting out on a road trip made life seem easy, more
normal. That was a misguided thought. It was not easy! And it
certainly wasn't normal to load a wheelchair, a walker, and a
portable commode into my SUV, amidst overloaded suitcases,
my computer, and a picnic cooler, but we did—and we set off.
And I am glad we did.

Betty and I shared the driving, and we never stopped talking.
David was in the back seat—quietly taking in the scenery, or so
I thought. When I asked him what he was doing, he simply
said, "Driving." I glanced at Betty with eyebrows raised. We
didn't say anything, but we were each worried. I stole glances
in the rearview mirror. Was David's mind so confused that
he actually thought he was driving the car? I questioned him
further. He said he was imagining how he'd maneuver through
traffic or take the turns. He calculated his speed as if he were
at the wheel. Phew! I sighed. David, my husband, the racer—
always the driver!

The trip let me share more of our country than just New
York City with Betty. The 450-mile drive to Erie, most of it along
the Southern Tier Expressway on the border between New
York and Pennsylvania, is beautiful. The word "expressway"

is deceiving. Yes, the road is a four-lane, high-speed highway, but once out of the reaches of New York City, it wends its way through the forests of the Catskill and Appalachian Mountains. It follows the Susquehanna River and crosses the Allegheny River. It passes through the Seneca Reservation and the Allegheny National Forest. Small towns stem off of the exits, with names like Kanona, Prattsburg, Horseheads, Gangs Mills, and Lounsberry. Unlike the hustle-bustle of traffic in the New York area, the drive is calm with little traffic, but at ten hours, it is still long. We stopped a lot for David—bathroom stops, stretch stops, and snack stops. But near the end, we were rewarded with a most beautiful view of Presque Isle on Lake Erie. Every time I see that stretch of blue, I know we are near home.

Hank's home, which was similar in style to David's and mine, looks out over a gorge—a peaceful, private, wooded area. I felt my stress slowly ebb as we unpacked our bags and settled in for the visit. I knew David and his dad would enjoy countless hours at the dining table in serious conversation—solving the problems of the world. It was their habit every weekend—long distance, courtesy of Ma Bell, before David's TBI. Their time together allowed me snatches of rest and free time, which I desperately needed.

But not too much rest—I was excited to share my hometown with Betty. No, it wasn't New York City. Erie is much smaller, definitely quieter, and runs at a snail's pace compared to New York. I took Betty, David, and Hank to the Peninsula on Lake Erie, and we walked around Perry Monument. Hank, with his bad knee, pushed David's wheelchair. He insisted it helped him walk. Betty and I walked along the shore of the lake gathering shells for my students. Before we left the beach, we stopped at Sara's for ice cream. Sara's is a small '50s-style restaurant, complete with a red-and-white 1957 Chevy and original coke machines haphazardly decorating the property. We never again went to the beach with Hank without stopping there.

We drove from one end of Erie to the other, pointing out our favorite spots, including Cathedral Prep where David went to high school and Villa Maria Academy, where I went. We drove by the church where David and I were married and past Y-Co, where we met. And we stopped each time I screamed, *"Frog!"* I've grown fond of frogs since I wrote the children's picture book manuscript, *School Is NO Place for a Frog*. I photographed every frog sculpture I saw. They were posed on street corners, in front of office buildings, stores, and restaurants. (The frogs were the result of a fundraiser that Erie sponsored in 2004.) It was fun showing Betty where David and I grew up. I wanted to test David's memory too, and I was relieved that he remembered everything.

One evening as David and Hank sat talking and watching the news, Betty and I slipped out to the mall. We headed to the ear-piercing studio. I wanted more piercings and would've gotten two more on each side, making a total of six piercings, but Betty insisted on only three—one on my right earlobe, two on the left. Five was fashionable, she insisted. So that's what I did. Who was I to defy fashion?

The next night I decided to get my nose pierced. I was on a roll—of insanity, some might think. I had to go to a special studio for the piercing. That brilliant idea was born when Kiersten visited in March. One day, as David lay napping in his room at Radburn, Kiersten announced that she and Treska planned to get their noses pierced. I looked at her incredulously and said, as any well-meaning mother would have, that she was out of her mind. If Kiersten were still my teenaged daughter and not the thirty-something-year-old daughter she was, I would've discouraged her from getting her nose pierced. Instead, I dared her. I said if she was going to get her nose pierced, so was I. She said, "Let's go!" And so, we went. Fortunately, the piercing studio was closed. Phew! I breathed a sigh of relief. Time ran out, and Kiersten returned to Taos unpierced, but the seed had been planted in me.

And so, when I was in Erie, I searched the Yellow Pages of the phone directory for a piercing studio. I found Ink Assassins, Mad Mike's, and Buddha's Body Art. Buddha's sounded the least scary, so Betty and I drove there. The piercing didn't take long—a cork up my nostril and a needle poke through the nose cartilage—*ouch!* Then the piercer slipped the cubic zirconium corkscrew piercing through my nose and voila! I had another hole in my head! A few moments later, I stood in the night under the pink fluorescent lights wondering what in the world I had done. It was creepy. But I'm glad I did it. David even liked it.

After showing Betty the highlights of Erie, including the Erie Zoo, we decided to venture farther. Since Niagara Falls is about a three-hour drive from Erie, we packed a picnic lunch and headed there for the day. The Falls, as we fondly call them, are amazing. I could never fully describe their magnitude and beauty, and I wanted Betty to experience them. I knew she'd be amazed. Who wouldn't be? As a child growing up in Erie, I picnicked at the Falls with my family nearly every summer. I never tired of the Falls' majesty, and I am still in awe of this natural wonder of the world. We picked the perfect day. Although it was hot, the misty spray from the Falls cooled us as we chomped on our peanut butter and jelly sandwiches under a shady tree. It was a lovely day, and Betty was excited to have her passport imprinted with the Canadian stamp.

Before we headed back to New Jersey, I had a few more hometown needs to fulfill and share with Betty. She had to taste my favorite, Pio's Pizza, and the delicious Lake Erie perch fish fry at Nunzi's. She loved them both. During this trip, Betty became a very important and special part of our family. She still is.

CHAPTER 30

An Invitation to Speak

We stayed in Erie for about ten days. I didn't do any other "crazy" things while there. But my best friend from Louisville came to visit on her way home from her parents' home in Buffalo. She and I can be crazy just doing nothing.

Patty Williams Streips, or Trish as I called her, was one of my dearest and oldest friends. (It greatly saddens me that she lost her battle with cancer in the spring of 2014. I miss her. It helps that through the years she gifted many trinkets to me. An Oil of Old Age lotion bottle, a frog that clings to my printer, and an angel coin we got in Estes Park are constant reminders of my friend.) Trish is not to be confused with my dear and older cousin, Patti Wunder Williams, who is also a friend. Though they share "Williams," the two never met.

When Trish called to tell me that she was passing by Erie on her way home from her folks' place in Buffalo, I was excited. We occasionally talked on the phone, and we emailed, but we did not often see each other, and I could not wait to spend time with her. I was anxious about her seeing David. She was not going to see the man she knew. I worried about her reaction, but Trish, as usual, was unflappable. It was as if nothing had changed—like old times.

"Hi, Dave, how are you?" she said as she wrapped her arms

around him in her customary hug. Then Trish and I were off to the front stoop to talk—and to laugh. I needed to laugh! When Trish and I were together, we never stopped laughing.

Trish and I first started laughing together in Rochester, New York, when David was a graduate student in the Department of Microbiology at the University of Rochester and she was a secretary in the department. We saw each other at department functions, picnics, and parties and became fast friends. Then one day, she unexpectedly announced that she was moving to San Diego. Her news crushed me, but soon after David accepted a postdoctoral position at the University of California at San Diego, and I was ecstatic to know my friend would be there too. Trish left before us and rented a house in Pacific Beach, just blocks from the ocean. In October 1974, David and I drove our Dodge van, packed fender to fender, across country with four-year-old Kiersten squashed in the back seat and unborn Jared in utero. When we arrived in San Diego, we drove straight to the ocean at Pacific Beach. I thought I was in heaven. Then we drove the few blocks to Trish's house and crashed there for a week until we found a nearby apartment to rent.

Trish lived in Pacific Beach for almost two years before she, with a lot of encouragement from me, moved to Louisville to be near her boyfriend, Uldis, a former postdoctoral scientist at Rochester. With Trish in Louisville, I missed her and our "girly giggly" times. When she was in San Diego and David attended an out-of-town scientific conference, she would stay with me. She became my roomie. Once my kids were in bed, we'd stay up half the night sipping wine and talking and laughing— laughing at everything and at nothing at all. I hated to see her move back East, but I knew it was best. Uldis was in love with her. He wanted to marry her, and I knew they were good together. They were married for nearly forty years.

I missed my friend when she moved from San Diego. The cross-country miles did not break our bond, though. I visited Trish and her family in Louisville many times through the years. One summer, Trish and I even met at Lake Erie to camp for a girl's week out. We "pounded" our stakes into the sand of the beach, just a few hundred yards from Sara's at the edge of Presque Isle. We arranged our door flaps only feet from each other so we could lean out and talk late into the night, and giggle too, of course. So Trish was no stranger to Erie, and we spent her visit doing what we do best—talking and giggling.

A few years ago, Trish sent me a picture of herself at a baby shower with her friends. I smiled when I looked at it. She was laughing hysterically. I sent her this email:

Hey Trish,

Cool pict. Thanks for sending it.

You were doing what you do best . . . laughing!

It made me laugh just to see you laugh. It's contagious, friend.

Love you.

Donna

She replied:

I laugh best when I am with you.

trish

Oh so true! So did I when I was with her!

We didn't get to laugh long enough on her very short visit in Erie. She still had a long drive home to Louisville. But before Trish left, Uldis called me with an astounding request. He asked if David would be the keynote speaker for the 2006 Wind River Conference on Prokaryotic Biology, a meeting that Uldis organized each year. He said that the conference, held near Estes Park, Colorado, was celebrating its fiftieth anniversary and he would be honored if David would accept the speaking engagement. Emotions flooded me. I was amazed. I was terrified. I was excited. I was proud, so proud, of my husband, who had the respect of esteemed scientists in his field.

This was an immense honor. To be honest, I didn't know if David could meet this challenge. I worried that Uldis didn't fully realize the severity of David's trauma. He couldn't know how David had become reliant on someone for his needs twenty-four hours a day, seven days a week.

I told Uldis that, although David's cognitive mind—and therefore his scientific brain—was in perfect order, David's brain injury had severely damaged his vocal chords and his speech was not easily understandable. Though David was learning to speak again, I was unsure he could perform as Uldis expected. Uldis reminded me that the conference was a year out and David had plenty of time to heal. He insisted that David be keynote speaker. He said that speaker commitments would be finalized in January 2006 and that, if David were uncomfortable about speaking or unable to make the trip, he'd understand and sadly fill the speaking slot with another scientist. With misgivings, I passed the phone to David, and he and Uldis sealed the deal. I don't believe that Uldis, even today, knows how critical his phone call was in restoring David's confidence to return to his scientific life.

Too soon, it was time for Trish to be on her way to Louisville, and it was with hugs and vows of love that she drove away. I waved and smiled knowing that we would be together in a year in Estes Park, where I knew our laughter would continue.

It was soon time for us to leave Erie too. Saying goodbye to Hank was difficult. David enjoyed the time with his father, and I enjoyed the false sense of freedom, but back to New Jersey it was. After nearly a four-month absence, I finally returned to my first grade classroom. I was excited to see my kiddles. I worried that they had bonded with their substitute teacher and had completely forgotten me, but I was wrong. Their affection for me remained strong. They were as excited to have their "real" teacher return as I was to be back with them.

During the next two months, Betty and David hung around the house. They ate breakfast and lunch together. Betty drove David to his therapy sessions at Radburn's Outpatient Department during the afternoons, and we both accompanied him to his evening appointments with his neurologist and optometrist. David's days were filled. He spent countless hours exercising. Though each therapist—physical, occupational, and speech—required *only* ten repetitions of each exercise, they each assigned at least five exercises. Do the math—fifteen different exercises.

David was in perpetual motion. He attempted to balance in the corner for his physical therapist. He stacked cubes for his occupational therapist. She also assigned a variety of eye exercises to strengthen his eye muscles to help him regain his vision. His speech therapist gave him what seemed like reams of pages of speech sounds to practice. David also included many of his favorite former exercises to his daily regime. His chores seemed endless, and it was exhausting for him to complete all of the exercises each day, but he met the challenge with no complaint.

It was a challenge for me to juggle my life too. My school day and my responsibilities at home seemed endless. I admit though, unlike with David, more than a few complaints slipped from my mouth. Having more than an hour and a half commute to and from school didn't help. Stopping at the grocery store to purchase the necessary ingredients for dinner each evening added to the stress of getting home, but I simply was not organized enough to have everything planned. I was living day by day. Minute by minute would be more accurate.

Sometimes Betty had dinner ready when I arrived, and I was grateful, but most times, I prepared it. I enjoyed it most when Betty and I joined in the kitchen to throw something together, but it wasn't easy. There were a lot of food restrictions. Betty was vegetarian, but she'd eat dairy. David was restricted to soft, mushy foods. Think applesauce or pudding. I needed to be creative to accommodate each of their needs. Some of our favorites were bean burritos or grilled cheese with tomato soup. Scrambled eggs or French toast was popular, though the latter is not very nutritious.

Betty's stay with us seemed too short. She and David spent countless hours together talking. They became close, and I knew he'd miss her. I would miss her too, desperately. I would lose a good friend and confidant and helper. I dreaded the day we'd drive Betty to the airport.

Much too soon, the day came. The drive across Manhattan and through Queens to the JFK Airport was hard. There was so little time to convey our deepest feelings before Betty departed to another world. We made promises to call and to write. Thank technology for email. She vowed to return, and we promised a trip across the ocean to Leipzig to see her when David was well enough to travel. Secretly, we each knew that would not be anytime soon. We hugged again and again—each with our separate thoughts. We didn't want to let go. A tear escaped and rolled down my cheek. I saw David discreetly wipe one away too. I told Betty I loved her, and she said, *"Ich hab dich lieb."* I tried to repeat it, but it got tangled on my tongue. David told her he loved her like a daughter. Then we watched her final wave as she passed through the security gate and disappeared down the long jetway to her plane. My tears unleashed. They streamed down my face as I wheeled David through the airport.

During the last weeks of Betty's stay, I arranged for David and me to go to California to be near our son, Jared. That thought alone held me together as we retraced our miles from the JFK Airport, across the George Washington Bridge to our very quiet, lonely home in New Jersey.

Before I agreed to make the trip to California, I made certain that David would get the medical attention he desperately needed. Jared located a small hospital in Santa Cruz, only two miles from his home. Though Dominican Hospital was reputed to have an excellent therapy department, I was skeptical. David was receiving outpatient therapy at Radburn. Its reputation was nationwide. I doubted a small, local hospital could equal Radburn's quality.

It was arranged that David would continue to receive Vital Stim therapy at another hospital. His doctor wrote a letter of medical necessity, insisting that David continue this remedy. So Jared searched for a facility to administer the treatment. VitalStim is a speech and swallow therapy in which six electrodes are applied to the patient's face and throat. Then a small measure of electrical current is delivered to stimulate the swallow nerves and muscles in the throat. Doctors believe that stimulation may reeducate the affected nerves and muscles and encourage them to return to their pre-trauma state. We tried anything.

In David's case, the intent was also to stimulate David's droopy facial muscles, which distorted the right side of his face. His facial paralysis not only interfered with his ability to chew, but it also led to his garbled speech. El Camino Hospital in Mountainview, California, more than an hour away, was the closest facility providing these services.

Though David's insurance policy didn't require precert-ification for medical services, Jared spoke with a representative to ensure that there would be no glitch in coverage. For extra measure, I called too. The representatives assured both Jared and me that the therapies David would receive at both Dominican Hospital and El Camino Hospital were fully covered.

I was eager to spend a partial summer in Santa Cruz. I was looking forward to the change of scene, and I was grateful for Jared's help. I was anxious too. Anxious, fretful, and beyond overwhelmed were three adjectives that strongly described me. I felt swamped as I searched for flights, arranged a car service to take us to and from the airport, and packed for a stay of four weeks while still managing everyday life, which was not "everyday" anymore.

Traveling with David was a mini nightmare. I had to juggle extra luggage, his computer, my computer, a carry-on bag, and my backpack while he was transported at warp speed through the airport by a wheelchair attendant. I lagged behind, panting. Both David and his wheelchair were searched extensively. Good thing we arrived at the airport early.

Once on the plane and seated near the front, I was calm. I relaxed until David had to use the restroom. His compromised bladder forced him to use the restroom often, and he used it several times during the cross-country flight. Fortunately, the attendant allowed him to use the first-class restroom, which was closest and easiest. The journey from our seats to the restroom was a challenge. David planted his hands on my shoulders as I slowly guided him down the aisle. With the plane's dips and jolts, it was a precarious trip. Imagine the stares. One young woman physically recoiled and glared at us. Did she think we were terrorists, this broken man and me?

The attendants were wonderful. They made the flight

comfortable for David and for me too. We shared stories as they prepared meals and I waited for David. In those early days of recovery, David easily would be in the bathroom for twenty minutes. His bladder sent urgent messages to his brain to use the toilet, but when he was there, his bladder rarely cooperated. It was a waiting game. Hence, I spent long minutes loitering outside of men's restrooms—receiving a good deal of questionable stares.

I was relieved when we disembarked at the San Jose airport and I saw Jared's smiling face. I was glad to share the burden, if only for a few weeks. Being near Jared, knowing that he understood the seriousness of our situation and that he deeply loved his father, as I did, comforted me. Since Jared's bungalow was small, Jared arranged for us to stay with his friends, Diana and Diego, in Davenport, about thirty minutes up the coast. Jared assured me numerous times that we were welcome in their home gratis. I was amazed by the California friendliness and generosity.

It was late. Our trip had been arduous. David and I were exhausted. We thanked Diana and Diego and bid good night. Jared promised to see us the next day. I unpacked only what we needed for the night. We'd move in in the morning.

Sometime after midnight, David and I crawled into bed, and I felt a release as we fell into an immediate deep sleep. I was sure nothing could wake me. I was wrong. About 4:00 a.m., a yell jolted me upright. I scrambled out of bed and ran to the bathroom. The toilet was gushing. Water flooded the bathroom floor and flowed into the kitchen. Apparently, David had fallen against the toilet and had broken the tank. I found him clinging to the kitchen sink. I never found out how he got from the bathroom to the kitchen, about five feet away, in just seconds. He wasn't able to move on his own, and his walker was still in the bathroom. It remains a mystery. David can't explain it either. He looked scared, like a child caught with his fingers in the cookie jar. He looked embarrassed too, and my heart broke for him.

How I knew what to do is still beyond me, but I sloshed through the water and turned off the valve behind the toilet. I didn't consciously know there was a water valve, but I guess in desperation my unconscious mind took over. Thankfully, the water stopped. I grabbed towels and started to mop up the river. I freaked out. I wanted to scream, to yell, but one look at David's panicked face squashed those feelings. My protective hormones kicked in. I led him back to the bed. I assured him that everything was okay, though I didn't believe it. I wished that we'd stayed home, that we'd never come. I thought I'd made a poor decision, and I was angry with myself for making an already difficult situation even harder. Everything was unfamiliar, and David had a hard time adjusting. At least at home he knew what to expect. I wanted to get on the next flight home, but I didn't. I called Jared for help—at four o'clock in the morning.

Jared brought a bucket loaded with towels and rags. He also brought his calm, patient manner, and he told me everything would be okay. He said he'd fix the tank. He'd make it right. I wasn't reassured. I was embarrassed, and I know David was too. Though Diana and Diego were amazing and told us not to worry, I can't help but wonder if they regretted their invitation. If they did, we'll never know. They were gracious hosts. The next day they invited us, Jared, and other friends to a Sunday brunch on their deck overlooking the Pacific.

The rest of the week passed uneventfully. I drove the coast road to Santa Cruz three mornings a week for David's therapy at Dominican. On those same days, we made the two-and-a-half-hour round trip over the mountain to El Camino Hospital for Vital Stim therapy. We spent a lot of time in our rental car. Each night we enjoyed dinner with Jared before trekking back to Davenport. When the week was up, we hugged Diana and Diego goodbye and thanked them with a ton of gifts for their home and their expected baby. Then we moved to Bill and Ali's house, also friends of Jared's, to housesit while they traveled Europe for three weeks.

CHAPTER 31

Open-air Gym

Bill and Ali were gracious hosts too. Though they were in the midst of home renovations, they welcomed us. They made a special effort to make us comfortable. They worked in the middle of the night before they left, which was the night before we arrived. As they finished packing their bags and completing last minute errands for their trip to Italy, they worked diligently to install a toilet on the second floor. There was a working bathroom on the first floor, but David couldn't use it at night. They also installed a railing on the stairway for David's safety. Bill and Ali did not get much sleep that night.

Their house was spacious, and that was good. David needed space to shuffle around on his walker. The floor was a beautiful, brand new hardwood, and I worried David's walker would gouge it. The rubber feet wore out quickly, so I attached tennis balls to the legs and double-wrapped them in old socks. This worked. No scrapes. No gouges.

Staying at Bill and Ali's house was convenient. It was centrally located in Santa Cruz and only minutes from the grocery store. Still, going to the market was tricky. It wasn't safe for David to stay home alone, and it was difficult for him to come into the store with me. It would have turned a fifteen-minute errand into an hour-and-fifteen-minute chore. We developed a system. He'd stay in the car with his phone at the ready, and I'd call every ten minutes to check on him. He was content as he patiently listened to a political talk radio station. My grocery trips were quick. I'd dash from aisle to aisle, grab what I needed for that night's dinner, and check out.

Bill and Ali's house was a convenient drive to Dominican Hospital too—only ten minutes away. Our mornings started early. Although David's sessions began at 9:00 a.m., his alarm rang at 6:30 a.m. It took him forever to shower, shave, eat breakfast, and get dressed. Routine morning activities, which before his brain injury took only an hour to execute, now took more than double that time. In fact, everything David did took an unbearable amount of time. I've learned patience—a virtue not generally attributed to me. I had to readjust. It was not easy.

David's therapy lasted until 12:00 p.m. It started with physical therapy. Mike was his therapist for two of the days. Mary Anne was responsible for one session a week. They were wonderful. I stayed for all the sessions, sitting on the mat with David as Mike or Mary Ann demonstrated each exercise and David executed them. Mike liked to put David on a treadmill, much like the one Jeff used at Radburn. It took a lot of time to attach the harness to David, but David got some good strengthening exercise with that machine.

The machine that cracked me up looked like a giant baby walker. I don't know its real name, but that's what I called it. Again, David was secured in a harness, which was attached to an overhead pole at the top of the machine. He pulled the contraption along the hospital corridors while Mike or Mary Anne followed behind. David was suspended, his feet barely brushing the floor. The purpose was to shift his weight so he could move one foot in front of the other, simulating walking. He looked like a marionette dangling from overhead strings, which, of course, made me laugh. That may sound cruel, but David laughed too. Laughter got us through many difficult days.

It was Mike's goal to improve David's ability to walk. And it was my goal to help David practice. Santa Cruz is at the edge of Monterey Bay—a beautiful place—and this haven made a wonderful outdoor gym. Just blocks from our borrowed home were the cliffs along West Cliff Drive. Each day hundreds of walkers, bicyclists, and skateboarders pass along the cliff's winding path overlooking the bay. David and I joined them on the days that he was not in the gym. Before David's brain injury, he'd run the length of the cliff trail to Natural Bridges State Park and back, totaling approximately five and a half miles. It took him about forty minutes. After the TBI, it took him forty minutes to hobble only a few hundred feet. But one very unbalanced step at a time brought him closer to his goal.

Most days, I left David's walker in the car, and I hung onto him—for dear life, literally! A short breeze could offset his balance and blow him over. David set his goals far. We walked about twenty minutes each way. It was hard work supporting him. I can only imagine how difficult it was for him, but no matter. We both trudged on.

One day as we were ending our walk, David made a misstep and stumbled, dragging me halfway down with him. So much for my thinking I could support him! Most of the cliffs were covered with ice plant, and the sheer drop to the bay was safely at a distance from the pathway, but at a few places, only a small fence separated the path from the steep drop-off to the bay. Of course, that is where David tripped. We each clutched at the fence to break our fall. I remember hoping it wouldn't break under our combined weight. I guess you could say we were literally living on the edge.

Where the cliff juts out and where the ice plant grows are dirt trails, and benches were placed along those paths. David and I took breaks on those benches to watch the sea otters frolic in the surf. A kelp forest hid under the waves off the shore, and the otters loved to play there.

David used the benches to practice balancing. He'd stand behind a bench, and I'd stand behind him. At my urging, he'd let go, wave his arms in the air, and twist his body from side to side. It sounds easy, but for someone with no sense of balance, it was a daunting task. I monitored him carefully. He swayed to the right. He leaned to the left. Sometimes he would drift backwards, and my slight touch would set him straight again. But once he lurched forward unexpectedly, and I nearly lost him. He went head first over the bench. This time we were far from the cliff's edge, so there was no danger of his falling into Monterey Bay, but it was scary just the same. We laughed, and our laughter shook us as we hugged.

We loved the cliffs, our open-air gym. We loved the blue, and sometimes gray, sky. We loved the music of the waves slapping the shore. We enjoyed watching the kelp swaying in the water and the sea otters slipping through it. We loved the way other trail walkers smiled or nodded to us or stopped to share encouraging words with us. But mostly we loved the way we laughed with abandon, briefly forgetting why we were there and grateful that we were.

We laughed one day when I innocently and proudly told Mike of David's great job balancing on the cliffs the day before. When I saw Mike's shocked look, I realized what I'd said. If therapists, like teachers, have the duty of reporting any suspected abuse of their clients to a service, such as the Division of Family and Youth Services (DYFS), then I think Mike's mind was whirring. *No! No! Not on the edge of the cliff!* "David was in no danger of falling into Monterey Bay," I added, and Mike looked relieved.

That incident reminded me of David's first Vital Stim appointment with Faye in New Jersey. Betty and I sat quietly as Faye rattled off a list of introductory questions. I answered most of them for David, but when Faye asked him if anyone hurt him at home, David quickly pointed at me and said, "Yes, she punches me!" Then he pointed at Betty and said, "And she beats me!" Betty's face went white. "No, I don't!" she protested. David suppressed a grin, and I laughed. Betty didn't. When I saw Faye's expression, I realized that this was serious. Just as I had to report suspected abuse of any of my students, I instinctively knew Faye did too. David was in a short-lived joking stage, which began as soon as he arrived home from the hospital. This behavior was so unlike the serious David from before his injury. Now he made a joke out of everything and kept his visitors entertained. I knew he was teasing, but Faye didn't.

I explained the ramifications of David's statements to him, and fortunately Faye realized that he was just being funny. She probably still reported it. If a child ever hinted at abuse to me, I would have to too. So I understood when Mike's face clouded over, ever so briefly, when I told him I had David balancing on the cliffs.

After Mike finished working David's large muscles, David spent an hour with Gillian working on strengthening his tongue and swallow muscles and practicing speech sounds. I didn't always stay for Gillian's sessions. Sometimes I used that time to write my book reviews, but I never wandered far. I needed to be near to help David to his next therapy area. He used his walker, but he wasn't steady on it, and his double and blurred vision made it difficult to see where floor surfaces changed. A doorway threshold could make him stumble.

The last session each morning, occupational therapy at 11:00 a.m., was the most enjoyable. David's wild-haired occupational therapist Terryn was amazing! Though she was scheduled to work with David until noon, she rarely stopped before 12:30—working through most of her lunch hour. I loved the time we spent with Terryn. She laughed with unleashed abandon, and we laughed heartily with her. Her laugh was loud, filled with joy, and carried across the gym. I often wondered what her fellow therapists thought. Terryn was new to Dominican Hospital, and I worried that she would fall out of favor with her administrators. This was a job . . . wasn't it? Terryn was having entirely too much fun.

Terryn was an out-of-the-box thinker and always devised new challenges for David. It didn't matter that she'd twist him up like a pretzel. Those funny contortions were intended to improve his fine motor skills and his balance while stretching and strengthening his muscles. Terryn loved to make David show off. "Ta-da!" both of them would say together as David surpassed yet another wild goal that Terryn had set for him. Terryn's dynamic personality and her passion and exuberance for her profession was a medicine all its own.

Terryn's exuberance spilled outside of the gym too. She visited us at our borrowed home on two occasions. Her visits were under the guise of "home evaluation," but really they were for Jared's freshly caught salmon, our disjointed conversations, and the quick-bonded friendship. Jared grilled the salmon. I tossed a salad, boiled corn, and set the table while David and Terryn put their heads together over David's laptop. They practiced the talk David would give at the Wind

River scientific symposium in Estes Park the following June. I expected she'd listen to ten minutes of his talk to be polite, but she listened to every last word, asking pertinent questions about the topic, showing David where to take breaths, and coaching his speech sounds. She was surprised by the solid grasp David demonstrated on his presentation and was amazed, as most people are, at his intellect. Terryn was one of the first people who helped David restore his confidence in himself as a scientist. She surpassed her duties as his occupational therapist. She became his friend and mine too.

On David's and my anniversary on August 9th, I made dinner reservations at the Crow's Nest on East Cliff Drive, a favorite restaurant of ours. Its beautiful view of the bay, the harbor, and the lighthouse is relaxing. Jared joined us on the outdoor patio. It was a lovely surprise to find a bottle of fine wine on our table. We thought Jared had arranged it. He thought we had. I eagerly reached for the card. It wished us a happy thirty-sixth anniversary and was signed by David's Dominican therapists. We were flattered.

Terryn told us the next day about her narrow escape. She'd asked the maître d' to put the wine on our table, and as she was leaving the restaurant, she saw our car pull into the parking lot. We were early. Terryn panicked. She dashed to her car and scrunched down beside the driver's door until we disappeared into the restaurant. Another reason to laugh.

CHAPTER 32

Definitely Not a Vacation

Our four weeks in Santa Cruz flew by. I was not ready to return home, and neither was David. I was nervous. To be honest, I was still anxious about being alone with my husband. Even in Santa Cruz, I was David's sole caregiver, but having Jared nearby was a welcome safety net. In New Jersey, I had no support. It was only the middle of August, and Kristin, a friend of a friend of Kiersten, wouldn't arrive until September. So, I did what any scaredy-cat would do: I extended our airline tickets for two additional weeks and made arrangements with both hospitals to continue therapies while Jared located another house-sit for us with other friends. This time we stayed at Steve and Rosie's house. Thank goodness for friends! Steve and Rosie's house was another perfect escape. But before we packed our bags and moved the few blocks from Bill and Ali's to our new temporary home, it was my turn for doctor attention.

Jared set up a contraption in the bathtub at Bill and Ali's to make it easier and safer for David to shower. He secured a rusty C clamp to the windowsill so David could easily grasp it as he climbed into the bathtub. It worked great for David, but it attacked me.

I knew it was there, so I felt really dumb as one morning I sleepily and mindlessly stepped into the tub and slammed my head straight into its edge. A nasty gouge bled profusely on my forehead. David heard my cry, but he couldn't help. He wasn't able to stand unassisted, so he was trapped in bed across the hallway. I carefully tugged on my pajamas, crept to the bedroom, collapsed on the bed, and waited for the bleeding to stop. After fifteen minutes and several blood-soaked towels, I panicked. David was scared too. We felt trapped. I needed to call Jared, and I gingerly reached for my cell phone on the bed stand and felt doubly dumb as I realized I'd left it on the kitchen table downstairs. I didn't want to go down the stairs because I knew any strain could increase the bleeding. So, we waited. Finally, the bleeding stopped—an hour later. After David had showered (without hitting his head on the clamp, which I then had triple-wrapped in towels), dressed, and devoured breakfast, we finally went to Santa Cruz Urgent Care. One glance at the rusty clamp convinced me that I'd need a tetanus shot, but I did not expect the stitches . . . two of them.

Extending our stay in Santa Cruz was good. David worked hard with his therapists, but his day was not over when we left Dominican Hospital around 12:30 p.m. He had another appointment at El Camino Hospital more than an hour away. At 2:00 p.m. David's therapist, Debbie, applied six electrodes to his face and throat for the Vital Stim treatment.

Three times a week, we trekked to El Camino Hospital. Much of the drive was beautiful. We wound through the redwood forest of the Santa Cruz Mountains on Highway 17 eating our peanut butter and jelly sandwiches. Sometimes we ate turkey or chicken sandwiches with mayo, but mostly we ate peanut butter and jelly. That was our lunch, our picnic in the car. The peanut butter and jelly sandwiches were messy, but they were what David wanted. He said they were easy to swallow. For the next eight years, he ate peanut butter and jelly sandwiches for lunch every day.

We made the return trip to Santa Cruz just in time to meet rush-hour traffic, but still we arrived by 5:00 p.m. at Five Branches Clinic of Traditional Chinese Medicine for David's last appointment of the day. At Five Branches, David's face, head, neck, arms, and feet were poked with nearly twenty acupuncture needles with the intention of arousing the nerves in his face and throat. We thought acupuncture might reawaken the nerves and prompt them to begin their normal, natural functions again. It's difficult to discern if either Vital Stim or acupuncture helped David. Neither offered a miracle. He remains plagued with swallow difficulties, and the right side of his face still droops, but we are left with the satisfaction that we tried, and with the possibility that time may still heal all.

During the six weeks that we stayed in Santa Cruz, many family and friends wished us well on our "vacation." Vacation? Was this a vacation? No! The Free Dictionary defines "vacation" as "a time of pleasure, rest, or relaxation." I agree with that definition, and I longed for a vacation. In California, a part of the definition might include whale watching. Well, we did see otters playing in the surf. Does that count? Reading a book while lying on the beach is a heavenly part of any great sun-and-surf vacation. Oops, no book, but we could *see* the sand while David practiced "balancing on the cliffs." A cruise! Everyone loves a cruise or a sunset sail. We could have sailed on the *Paragon*, the research boat Jared piloted. No need! With David's imbalance, he didn't need to board a boat. He felt like he was always on one. Vacation? There was no pleasure. There was no rest. There was definitely no relaxation. If that was a vacation, I never want one.

Those therapy days were long. Three times a week we kept that schedule. By 8:00 p.m., when dinner was finally over and the dishes put away, it was time for David to get ready for bed. Taking his pills, brushing his teeth, and getting into his pajamas took an hour at least. But we could sleep in the next day, then go "balancing on the cliffs" while enjoying our California "vacation."

Before we returned to New Jersey, Terryn visited once more. A little more salmon, a lot more giggling, and then it was time to say goodbye. I gave her earrings, which matched mine—a remembrance. She gave me two frogs holding each other. She knew I loved frogs. Fric and Frac, they were called. "Donna and David," she said. It was a tearful goodbye. We hugged. We promised to email, and we have. But I miss her. I miss her love for life. I miss her support. I miss her laughter. We promised to visit again. She spent several days with us in New Jersey in November of 2007, and we visited her in Santa Cruz in 2010. I don't know when our next visit will be, but I wish I could laugh with her again.

CHAPTER 33

Kristin

We boarded the plane to New Jersey on September 2nd with mixed emotions. I knew we'd miss living near Jared, sharing daily conversations and dinners with him, and the sense of security that he offered. We'd miss David's lighthearted but incredibly competent Dominican Hospital therapists, and we would definitely miss the California lifestyle. I was not eager to return to the rush of daily life in our New York suburb with too much traffic, too many people, and incessant noise, but we were eager to return home to things familiar. And we looked forward to meeting Kristin.

Kristin arrived from Leipzig shortly after we returned. In the short drive with Kristin from the airport to my home, I knew we'd love her. She was bubbly and confident. She was energetic and excited to be in the States. I was happy that she was joining our family for the next three months. She fit in immediately.

As we had done with Betty, we decided to squeeze in a trip to Erie. We drove to Erie before I returned to school. It was crazy. We had only a few days, but David wanted to see his father again. My mother, who lived in Phoenix, was in Erie visiting my sister and her husband. My mother hadn't seen David since before his trauma and wanted to, and we were glad to see her too. Once she returned to Phoenix, we didn't know when we'd get the chance to see her again. So, the decision was made. Kristin and I loaded up my Mazda Tribute, and we set off, retracing the route we took with Betty only three months earlier.

We did many of the same things with Kristin—the walk around Perry Monument and a quick beach walk to gather shiny water-worn stones for my new students. Kristin posed with the new frogs we found around town. We ate on the bay at Rum Runner's, and we had our favorite perch and pizza dinners. They were an easy few days, and they were fun, but still they were not a vacation.

We returned home late on September 7th, and I dragged myself out of bed the next day and made it to school on time for opening-day teacher meetings. David and Kristin went to therapy at Radburn Rehabilitation Center and Blum Hospital as we settled into a routine life—as if any of this life was routine.

The next week, David went to the Department of Microbiology's retreat. This was the retreat that David had organized the year before. It was the same one he worried about in March, while he was still an inpatient at Radburn. Kristin and I went with him on the first night. After we got David settled in the conference auditorium, we briefly listened at the door, but those scientists speak a foreign language. "Prokaryotic," "glycosylation," "actinomycetemcomitans," and "operon" were some of the words that leaked out of the room. It sounded like secret codes. We understood nothing! We went to the reception room to chat and chomp on cookies.

After each session, we met David and escorted him to the restroom—supporting him on each side. His bladder refused to function properly, and a scheduled restroom visit every two hours left him feeling more secure. Sadly, I was unable to attend the meeting the following day. Kristin and David had a good time without me anyway, and Kristin enjoyed meeting David's students.

Like Betty, Kristin took the bus to New York City on weekends. She loved the City. She visited all five boroughs and explored the museums. She liked to walk the streets downtown just to watch the city life. Some of her favorite areas were Greenwich Village, East Village, Soho, Little Italy, and Chinatown. She said she was hooked on Broadway, and every weekend she found herself in another theater. She saw *Lion King, Gypsy, 42nd Street, Chicago, Phantom of the Opera, Thoroughly Modern Millie, Wicked, Rent, Little Shop of Horrors*, and *Mama Mia*. She saw *Mama Mia* twice. I totally understand. What a great show! I planned to see *Mama Mia* again too. Kristin probably saw more shows in her short time here than David and I saw in more than twenty years of living near the City. I was a tad jealous, but also glad that she had the chance to experience them.

Some years later, I emailed Kristin and asked what she liked best about living with us. She wrote:

What a question! Everything I did with you was special for me, because it was unique. I just think of our daily dinners (we were sitting and talking and laughing . . .), the afternoon after Thanksgiving when we ate all the left over cookies, our DVD-evenings, the evenings when we all were on the computers playing a game (Snood). Then the day we visited Donna's workplace and David's. Just the fact that you let me be a part of your life is special for me. I got to know so many family members. Everybody was so nice. You made the three months unforgettable for me. You took me to so many places. I can just say, "Thanks."

She added:

The time I spent with you was just great. I just can say you are two wonderful people. You are openhearted, honest, frank, and very kind. I got to know you at a time that was very hard for you. I was amazed at how you dealt with the situation. Even when it was a hard time, you made always the best of it and didn't lose your humor. You gave me so much and I hoped I could help out and could support you.

And she did help. David and Kristin spent countless hours together. They fell into a daily schedule.

Instead of picking David up in front of the house for the drive to therapy, she walked him to his car, which was parked in a lot a block away. This provided an extra ten minutes of intense exercise for David. Kristin had no intention of making life easy for him. By challenging David, she'd actually make it easier in the days to come. When Kristin arrived in September, David's wheelchair was prominent in his life, but he soon traded it for a walker. By the time Kristin left, David had his sights on the four-pronged cane.

It was another teary time in another airport that November day when Kristin boarded her flight to Leipzig. How had the time passed so quickly? It seemed she'd only arrived. I wanted her to stay with us forever. She promised to visit again.

CHAPTER 34

Parade of Helpers

Kristin's departure left me scrambling for caregivers for David. He couldn't be left alone, and I was teaching until the December break. In the following weeks, we had a parade of company.

Kiersten, Treska, and Kaya were the first. They stayed a week. Looking forward to their visit eased the pain of missing Kristin. Then my brother John and his wife Carol stayed with us—our PP pals. In another lifetime, we would have met them at Phoenix's airport to enjoy the four-hour, nonstop-chattering drive to Puerto Peñasco for a little Mexican fling. Now we were happy enough to have them visit us in cold, dreary, snow-laden New Jersey. No sun, sand, or sea, but still the happy camaraderie.

John loved helping David with therapy. He had an edge on it, since he was working with his own son who was in a similar state as David. John coached David as he staggered up and down the hallway using only a four-pronged cane. David became steadier under John's watch.

Lastly, the week before my holiday break, my twenty-four-year-old niece from Michigan, Caitlin, came. She is my lovely goddaughter. We always hoped that she would spend some weeks with us as she grew up, but they were empty wishes. Now in a less-than-perfect time, she arrived, and I was delighted.

Obviously nervous, Caitlin said she was apprehensive and worried that she couldn't handle her uncle's altered state. He looked and sounded different. His voice was still garbled. She was afraid he wouldn't know her. But her fears faded moments after they reunited and he gave her a great big hug. Caitlin later told me with a giggle, "Uncle Dave is the same old Uncle Dave." They spent many hours together that week enjoying each other's company. It was wonderful to see our family. Each of them gave us the greatest Christmas present ever—the gift of their precious time when David and I needed it most.

When the Christmas holiday arrived, David and I again boarded a plane. Our destination was Taos, New Mexico, to spend the holiday with Kiersten and her family. Jared flew from Santa Cruz to meet us. David and I stayed at the house of Kiersten's friend Julie, which was across the dirt road from Kiersten's house. It wasn't only convenient, it was beautiful. Our view of the surrounding mountains, set under an endless sky by day and millions of twinkling stars at night, was breathtaking. Julie's home had a quaint cobblestone brick floor that shifted under each footfall, making it feel as though we were in a funhouse at Coney Island. It was fun for me, but for David, who was fighting a balance distortion, it was a wobbly world. He never complained. I worried for both of us and shadowed his every step.

Christmas morning at Kiersten's was a relaxing, lazy time sipping coffee, curled on the couch with nothing more to do than enjoy each other's company. We took hours opening presents. We *oohed* and *aahed* as each present was pulled from its colored wrapping. The morning stretched into late afternoon. Of course, Treska and Kaya each modeled their new shirts, sweaters, and skirts for us. By four o'clock, as the sun dipped behind the mountains, Jared and Falko escaped into the kitchen to prepare dinner. Sushi—about thirty rolls. So colorful! They were stuffed with red and green peppers, carrots, and avocado. They were too beautiful to eat, but eat them we did, every last one. Yum!

A highlight of our Taos trip, besides hanging out with our granddaughters, was meeting Ian T. Simms. Ian, then twenty-nine years old and a native of Taos, suffered a traumatic brain injury when a truck he was a passenger in crashed, rolled, and pinned him underneath. He was fifteen. Ian recounts his story in his book called *High Flight—An Extraordinary Survival Story*. David enjoyed the hours he spent with Ian comparing injuries and recoveries. Ian gave David hope. He was a strong, determined young man who set his goals high—to fly a plane again, which he did.

On our return home, we stopped in Phoenix. We stayed with my brother John and his family. It was our first time seeing our nephew, Little John, since he'd suffered his TBI only three weeks before David. David and Little John sat for hours discussing their fates, comparing their disabilities, and promising that they would fight to get better and do anything necessary to return themselves to their pre-trauma states. It was sad to see them as they sat at the kitchen table, both talking in their distorted voices. I fought the tears welling in my eyes, but their determination heartened me. Both of those men had a slim chance to live, and yet they were talking—distorted talking but talking nonetheless. They were alive, full of life, and they would get better. They had to!

CHAPTER 35

Angela

We spent a lot of time on planes as David recuperated. As we headed home after a nice holiday with family, we looked forward to meeting Angela, another young woman from Leipzig. We'd arranged for our flights to arrive around the same time in Newark. It was reassuring to see her smiling face as we entered the baggage area. We hugged. She stayed with David as I searched for our bags.

The airline made me hunt. It seemed they simply could not keep track of canes or walkers. The attendant sent me to the oversized baggage claim. The oversized-baggage claim agent sent me to the agent at the lost-baggage counter, who immediately returned me to oversized baggage. An hour later, and with no apologies, the lost-baggage attendant was convinced that the cane and walker hadn't arrived. I felt frazzled and lost myself. How would David negotiate our house without aids? Fortunately, the attendant noticed my exasperation and gave us replacements. She promised that David's cane and walker would be delivered as soon as they were located.

I wondered what Angela thought of me in those first hours. I was crazed, running from counter to counter. In between, I checked on David and Angela and reported my frustration.

David seemed calm enough, and he and Angela spent valuable time together.

Unlike Betty's and Kristin's visits, my school schedule didn't allow for any diversion trips with Angela. No Erie! I was disappointed because I wanted to show her new places too. She saw much of New York City on her own. She took a bus to the City every weekend. Like Betty and Kristin, she visited museums. The Museum of Modern Art and the Metropolitan Museum of Art were two of her favorites. She said she spent time in Soho and Tribeca, and she fell in love with Coney Island. Angela said, "I could sit on the boardwalk the whole day, watching the seagulls, the people, and the ocean." She saw two Broadway shows, *Stomp* and *Chicago*, and a lot of off-of-Broadway productions.

Though we hadn't planned to travel to Erie, fate had its way. In early February 2006, we received a dreaded phone call from David's father. David's Uncle Stan had died. It wasn't a surprise. We had spoken to his wife, Aunt Marie, only days before. She told us of Uncle Stan's deterioration. He was in the advanced stages of cancer and in excruciating pain. Death was inevitable. Still, it was a shock to hear he'd passed. He was the jokester in the family—always laughing, ever a smile on his face. Uncle Stan's gone, but our memories of him are not.

David insisted on going to his memorial. He is the oldest nephew. We went into overdrive. We packed. I wrote plans for my substitute teacher and emailed them to school. Then we jumped into the car for the long trek to Erie.

Traveling to Erie in mid-winter is scary. On any day, you can expect snow on the ground, falling from the sky, or on its way. It's always in the forecast. We were lucky on that trip. It only rained.

David donned his sport coat and slacks to go to the funeral

home. He hadn't dressed up in more than a year, and he looked handsome and *almost* normal. David's extended family had not seen him in his "trauma" state. Though Uncle Stan, in his coffin, was the silent star of the evening, David was the breathing one. His uncles, aunts, and cousins fawned on him.

Though time didn't allow a side trip to Niagara Falls, we did show Angela many of our favorite haunts. She got the fifty-cent tour of Erie—including Perry Monument along the bay and the beach. We ate my favorite fish and pizza, and photographed more frogs.

Once home again, we settled into a routine. David continued his therapy three times a week. Angela drove him to his sessions. Angela and David spent a lot of time together, much of it in political discussion, a topic they both enjoyed. They listened to books on CD and worked side by side on their computers. David made steady progress in his rehabilitation, and though advances were small and agonizingly slow, we embraced even the most minute progress.

David used the four-pronged cane exclusively. He became relatively independent in the house. He was self-sufficient in showering, shaving, getting dressed, tying his shoes, dispensing water from the refrigerator door, and getting his own vitamins and pills. It may sound silly to be enumerating seemingly menial tasks, but these were milestones. Of course, it took him three times—no, four times—as long as it did pre-trauma to accomplish these deeds. Considering his limited independence when he first arrived home from Radburn and for many months after, these accomplishments were very welcome!

Sometimes David made attempts to walk without his cane, using the hallway walls as bumpers. He bounced off them to retain balance. (Think pinball machine.) I watched and held my breath. Sometimes I laughed. It was a sight. Often I smiled and

marveled at how far he'd traveled in just one year, and how far
he had yet to go. His determination, persistence, patience, and
his firm desire to be well again will prevail. My husband is an
amazing man! I knew that the moment I met David when I was
sixteen, and I've never wavered in my belief. Okay, he wasn't a
man then—just a boy—but I knew.

David continued to practice walking outside each day as
well. His goal was to tackle the street unassisted. In the early
months, David clung to his walker with Betty on one side and
me on the other. We hung onto him for dear life. It was not
easy, not for any of us. Though walking unaided continued to
challenge David a year after his trauma, he was steadier. With
Angela and me and no walking device, he'd walk a respectable
distance down the street, about four city blocks. Of course, we
flanked him, ever ready to provide support, but usually a gentle
touch on his arm provided balance. It was an arduous process,
and baby steps and frequent rest stops—about eight—turned
the fifteen-minute walk into an hour-long trek. With much
practice and more time, David mastered the distance with only
one stop. Proof he was getting stronger!

Some days he'd stumble down that same street, looking as
though he'd had a drink too many, which, of course, he hadn't.
He avoids alcoholic drinks because they burn his throat, and
they don't mix well with his medications.

At the end of each walk, David had to make a right turn into
our driveway. He hadn't yet mastered the right turn. Frankly,
he hadn't mastered any turns. He once likened this task to an
albatross landing. Though I'd never seen an albatross land,
David's visual cracked me up. Believe me, his right turn was
not a pretty sight! Seriously, though, he was and is making
progress, and he provides fodder for laughter.

David continued to be plagued by swallow disorder. In early 2006, I took him to a swallow disorder specialist, which was a real joke—a costly mistake. The specialist used a new device, a tiny camera that revealed no more than what we already knew—that the right side of David's swallow mechanism remained paralyzed. And for our $1,700, David was the guinea pig! An inexperienced young doctor performed the procedure. She had obviously never done it before. David gagged as she practiced threading the endoscopic tube down his throat. She threw nervous backward glances at her mentor, who showed no concern that his student's unpracticed ministrations caused David undue pain.

And for his pain, David was advised to eat Level One— pureed foods with the consistency of pudding. The young doctor demonstrated the proper firmness as she stabbed a spoon into a cup of Jell-O. She said it must be freestanding and suggested foods like omelets, scrambled eggs, egg salad, or oatmeal as his daily fare. Not a varied diet! I held back tears. We'd come to this specialist with expectations and optimism, and our hopes were dashed. This was a step backwards.

I told the doctor that David had been cleared to eat Level Four (chopped foods) before he left Radburn at the end of March 2005 and that he'd been eating that food consistency for a year with no apparent problem. The doctor scoffed and arrogantly said he hears that from *all* of his patients. Then he smugly guaranteed that the next time he'd see David would be on a patient floor in a hospital if David didn't follow his prescribed plan of mushy foods.

I was overwhelmed. I felt inadequate, stupid, and guilty. How could I possibly have been so foolish to have served David chopped food? Was I setting him up for his demise? Had

Radburn been wrong? Was I gambling with David's life, as the doctor had proclaimed? I didn't think I was, and I still don't. We fled the doctor's office and his contemptuous ways.

That unwanted news threw a wrench in our afternoon plans. David and I had planned to take Angela to see his lab and then to lunch to presumably eat Level Four—chopped food. But eating was the last thing I wanted to think about. Yet it was the first and only thing on my mind. What could David eat? Not only for that day's lunch, but also for all his meals? I pondered those thoughts as we wended our way through the maze of hospital corridors to the mezzanine outside of the cafeteria in the Millstein building of Columbia-Presbyterian. That was not my original lunch destination, but I needed to think, and it was the only place nearby where we could sit and discuss this new discovery.

David was feeling down, understandably so, and he could not face going to a restaurant. Neither could I. We had looked forward to going to this specialist, hoping to improve David's eating situation, but now we were thrust back to square one. David refused to change his eating patterns. He continued taking small bites, did his chin tuck to the right, and took every precaution that he had been doing for the past year. He vowed never to return to that physician again, and I agreed.

Then I grabbed a couple of sandwiches from the cafeteria. David gingerly ate his. Angela devoured hers because it was way past lunchtime. I was unable to look at food. When David and Angela finished, I tossed their trash, and with it I flung out the disturbing feelings of the morning. Enough wallowing! Then we set off for David's lab and later for a meeting with Aaron Mitchell, his friend and the acting department chairman.

CHAPTER 36

Returning to Work

I watched with joy as David inserted his key into his office door. The key in his right hand wiggled for about a minute before it finally made contact and threw open the bolt. I offered no help. This was David's turf—his life—long lost. He was fighting to recapture it. I caught my breath as he walked through the door into the office that he had not seen in more than a year. Nothing had changed. It remained as it was the night he had left it on January 12, 2005. I wondered what thoughts raced through David's head. Was he remembering the life he had loved, his normal twelve-hour days as he guided the work of his graduate students and the research of his postdoctoral scientists? Was he remembering a time before time stopped, before life sent us hurtling down an unexpected and unwelcome path? I certainly was.

Fortunately, David's lab group continued their research and kept David involved. They met with him in his hospital room in the early months. When he returned home, they crossed the bridge to New Jersey for lab meetings in our living room. Over a year after his trauma, David planned to return to his lab two days a week as a volunteer. He wanted to be a steady presence in his lab group's lives. Because the lab group kept up with its work, this transition was easier.

Since November 2005, David's department chairman, Aaron, was in phone and email contact with both David and me sorting out the needs and details that would ensure David's smooth return. Aaron wanted to secure a part-time secretary to take dictation, type email, and type David's papers for publication. He secured an oversized computer monitor to make reading easier. (Actually, Saul Silverstein donated that, but I don't think David or I were supposed to know.) Nearly everything was in place, and David and I, with Angela in tow, went to Aaron's office to finalize the details.

David's first "practice" day back to work was March 7, 2006. He was welcomed, not only by his colleagues, but by Dr. Gerald Fischbach, Columbia's Vice President for Health and Biomedical Sciences and Dean of the Medical Center. David's interview, complete with photo, was published in the April/May 2006 issue of *In Vivo: The Newsletter of Columbia University Medical Center*. What an honor!

The Columbia University Human Relations office informed me that David was setting new precedents and they didn't know how to handle his type of paperwork. No one who had suffered a serious brain injury and been on disability so long had ever returned to work. David was charting new waters. He wasn't yet on Columbia's payroll. His return was a trial. We weren't sure if he had the stamina to tackle his tasks, but he was eager to try.

David also attended a student's PhD thesis defense that day. It was a busy first day. He came home exhausted, but he was exhilarated and eager to return on Friday for the weekly seminar. David continued a Tuesday and Friday schedule until September 2006, when he returned to work full-time. On the days that he didn't go to Columbia, David worked from home. He also went to Radburn for physical, occupational, and speech therapies. It was an exhausting schedule, but he did it with no complaint.

CHAPTER 37

Monique

Angela drove David to Columbia each day and accompanied him to his seminars. But at the end of March 2006, she needed to return to Germany. As I drove Angela to Newark Liberty International Airport, I was already anticipating Monique's visit with us.

It's funny—I never would've guessed I'd like having these young women live with us. I can't believe David agreed to it. We enjoyed our privacy, but having them share our home, being a part of our lives as we were in theirs, was comforting, and it was fun—well, as much fun as those days could possibly be. The chats around the dinner table brought us together each night to share stories, to solve problems, and to laugh.

Those dinners were the glue that held us together—and Angela agreed. When I emailed her to ask about her favorite experience with David and me, she wrote:

Having dinner together. No kidding—I loved our evening talks!

She continued:

In your house, I felt so at home and comfortable . . . and I loved your electronic can-opener. The "American time" became a very important episode in my life and I often talk with friends about my experiences in the States.

But her friends were most astounded when she told them of our TV-free home. Angela said:

Nobody here (Leipzig) believes me that I met an American family who lives without a TV.

It was a quick goodbye at the airport with Angela. Her flight and Monique's flight overlapped. After I waved goodbye to Angela, I greeted Monique with a hug. We stuffed Monique's luggage into my car, and we started to chat—first about her flight, then about her expectations for her life with us in America. Monique is an occupational therapist from Leipzig. She had recently completed the first phase of her degree and was eager to try out her profession on David. He'd be her guinea pig. I was excited to have Monique spend the next three months with us. She seemed to be a perfect fit.

As Monique walked up the stairs to greet David, her eyes roved over him. In an instant, she assessed him, seeking ways to improve his life. Her eyes sparkled in excitement, and when she smiled, I noticed a twinkle behind her top lip. Before she made it to the top step, I asked what it was. She smiled again, and I saw a small, diamond-like jewel resting against her top teeth. I'd never seen that before. It was pretty. It glittered and made her face light up. (I wanted one, but I am ahead of myself.) Monique fit into our little family instantly. She was bubbly and fun to be with. I knew we'd enjoy her living with us.

My spring break, coincidentally, happened the week after Monique arrived, and as you've probably already guessed, we stuffed the car with essentials to make the ten-hour journey to Erie to visit David's father. He'd never had so many visits from us in any prior 365-day period. Hank loved our visits, and he loved meeting the young women who were living with us. They loved him too. Many of the women kept in contact with Hank through postcards.

We did the usual things in Erie . . . and one not so usual. I was fascinated with Monique's sparkly jewel, and I had to have one. So, we searched the internet for a piercing studio. I'd never considered piercings beyond the normal ear adornments and my one nose piercing, but I was obsessed. I scoured Erie's Yellow Pages and found Ink Assassins. I didn't go there last year for my nose piercing because the name was scary, but it was nearby, and our time in Erie was running out.

Though I had suppressed my fear of the studio's name, Monique and I still circled the block again and again as I summoned courage. I was nervous. When we finally parked, I slammed the car door, took a breath, and together we pushed open the studio door. Missy, a piercer who seemed proficient with her craft, greeted us. Though she had *never* seen an upper lip frenulum piercing, which pierces the webbing under the top lip, she assured me she could do it. I trusted her. Unfortunately, she did not have the jewelry, and I had to abort the plan.

When we arrived home in New Jersey at the end of the week, I decided to leave David at home by himself for a few hours. Since he returned to his lab in March, he was comfortable being by himself for extended periods of time. We still kept each other on speed dial. Monique and I day-tripped to the East Village in Manhattan to a place called Venus Modern Body Arts. My apprehension was mixed with relief and disappointment when we found the store closed. But Monique reminded me we hadn't come this far to meet defeat. We searched for another studio— up one street and down another until we were completely lost in the maze of New York City streets. Some hours later, and purely by accident, we found ourselves in front of Venus again. This time it was open.

I leaned into the door, held my breath, and wondered why I was intent on putting myself through this pain. I mean, how stupid! Monique and I took our time picking out the prettiest gem. Looking at every tray—some twice. Finally, when I could delay no longer, I clenched my fists, climbed onto the chair, and scrunched my eyes. When it was over, I looked into the mirror and smiled. It was worth it.

I wonder if my three piercings—nose, ears, and upper frenulum—have any correlation to David's three brain surgeries. Hmmm. Well, I know I won't intentionally put any more holes in my head. My piercing days are over. I hope David will not tackle any more surgeries on his brain either.

With Monique's arrival, we moved into a new stage of David's development. He continued his appointments at Radburn three days a week for various therapies. Monique drove him. While there, she became friendly with David's therapists and some of the patients. She studied how American therapists did their jobs and was surprised and disappointed that the patients didn't receive continuous one-on-one therapy as they did at her place of learning in Germany. David's therapist would introduce an exercise—maybe leg lifts—and instruct him to do three repetitions of ten. Then he'd rush to the next patient to get him or her started on an exercise (e.g., a bike exercise or a leg press). He would then dash off to yet another patient to start him or her on something else. Finally, the therapist would return to David to guide him on his next exercise, and the procedure was repeated.

This service, divided by three patients, only provides actual patient-therapist contact of at most twenty minutes. How can a therapist assess a patient's needs and make the corrections to better rehabilitate a patient if the therapist is not physically working continuously with him or her? If a patient were receiving a full hour of attention, the patient might be rehabilitated more quickly. Something's wrong here!

I assured Monique that not all therapy facilities operated this way. I told her of Dominican Hospital in Santa Cruz, where David received six weeks of outpatient therapy. I told her the therapists at Dominican were amazing. They gave every minute of the hour and more to David. They studied, assessed, and readjusted his every movement to give him the best range of movement possible. How I wish we could have stayed there indefinitely, but school was opening in September for more "reading, writing, and 'rithmetic" for my first graders. I needed to be there with them.

David had commitments too. On the days David didn't have therapy, Monique went to the lab with him. Columbia provided a car service to pick up David twice a week. Once they even sent a stretch limo, which excited Monique. She took pictures to show to her friends back home. David enjoyed returning to work, if only for two days a week. This was a huge step in his campaign to regain his old life.

On the days that David stayed home, Monique worked her magic on him. She directed him through a variety of both large and small motor exercises. Picking up marbles, balancing on an exercise ball, walking up and down stairs, and simply putting one foot in front of the other with some semblance of balance were some of the challenges she presented to him. They went for walks through the neighborhood, and she even took him to the grocery store, where he pushed the cart up and down the aisles. Slowly but with determination, he did it. Monique never let up. Daily she dreamt up new goals for David, and he did his best to meet her demands.

One hellacious, stormy night as David, Monique, and I sat talking long after dinner, Monique showed us a picture she had drawn of a hummingbird and said she had to have it tattooed on her hip—right then! Though David and I looked skeptical,

Monique was insistent. I laughed and said, "Let's go." We hopped into the car and drove to a body-art studio in the next town. Her hummingbird was adorable. She tried to coax me to get one too. I refused. But imagine my surprise the next morning when I woke with a burning desire to get a hummingbird to match Monique's. Again we headed to the body-art studio. An hour later, Monique and I had twin hummingbirds. Mine adorns my chest. It's our personal connection. It's also proof that I didn't do crazy things only with Betty.

Some years later I asked Monique to remember her time with us and tell me what she thought. She had lots of nice things to say about her time in the City and visiting Niagara Falls and Erie, but the end of her email gives you a good idea of the kind of person Monique is:

For me, David and you are the strongest persons I ever met in my life! You're the best examples of how love should be, also in difficult times in your life. It showed me again what is really important when I have to make a decision. It doesn't matter if it is a decision for my work and my patients or for my own life! I'm a person who wants to plan everything and who wants to control everything that happens to me, but since I'm back in Germany that really changed. I'm still planning, but I'm not irritated if some things don't work. Thank you!

Hab dich ganz doll lieb!

Your hummingbird

You can see why I love this girl.

CHAPTER 38

Rocky Look-alike

Though more than a year had passed since David's trauma, his vision remained greatly impaired. It was still blurry, double, and tilted. His was a murky world. At home, David used a large monitor attached to his laptop and increased the font to make reading easier. His home monitor was not as large as the one in his office, but it was sufficient.

Vincent R. Vicci Jr, OD, PA, David's optometrist, suggested eye surgery to improve David's vision. We hoped for a miracle. (We *always* hoped for miracles!) With much anticipation, we set off to midtown Manhattan to the office of Mark Steele, MD, an ophthalmologist, to determine if David was a good candidate for the surgery. Dr. Steele explained the procedure, showed us pictures of his successes, and offered refreshed hope. We set a date in May 2006.

As the date approached, David and I both felt nervousness, fear, and excitement. Eye surgery is scary, but Dr. Steele assured us that the prescribed operation was less dangerous than cataract surgery. His goal, he said, was to balance David's ocular muscles and rid him of double vision. He hoped that David would need only a magnifier lens for reading and a slight prism prescription for distance vision. He explained that the procedure was painless. Though we dreaded the operation, we looked forward to it too and anticipated a positive outcome. If David could conquer this affliction, it would offer encouragement—one less roadblock.

On May 25th, we arrived early at New York University Hospital. David was soon gowned, prepped, and whisked off to surgery. He didn't see my tears as I watched the orderlies wheel him down the corridor. Déjà vu! Memories of his January 2005 surgeries engulfed me. How could I send him to surgery again? My comfort this time was his signature on the dotted line. When the operating door swung shut, I walked to the waiting room and waited with Monique.

After what seemed like forever but was only hours, Dr. Steele appeared. As he approached, I searched his face for signs that the surgery was successful. It went well, he told me, but David was still unconscious. The anesthesia had a grip on him. Dr. Steele warned me, as he led me to the recovery room, that David would not be a pretty sight. I peered into each cubicle of post-operative patients searching for David, and I cringed to see so many bruised faces. But their wounds did not prepare me for the pitiful sight of my husband.

The expected recovery room time for this surgery was about forty-five minutes. David must not have gotten the memo. He took several long hours to recuperate. I stood by quietly and watched him sleep. His face looked like it had a date with a meat grinder. Remember *Rocky II*? Sylvester Stallone said, "Was ya ever punched in the face five hundred times a night?" David looked like he'd been in the ring, and he was not the victor. Dr. Steele said this was normal. He gave me his personal email and his direct cell line and told me to call at my slightest concern. Healing would be slow.

More hours passed before David regained consciousness enough for Monique and me to stuff him into his clothes, prop him into the wheelchair, and make the journey across Manhattan and through the Lincoln Tunnel in five o'clock-rush-hour traffic—no easy feat. I am not, and never will be, a New York City driver. The trip terrified me, but I did it. One more hurdle jumped in this marathon called surviving traumatic brain injury—and not just for the victim.

When we arrived home, I put David to bed with his various painkillers and hoped that the morning would be better. But when the sun rose, though some of the pain had subsided, David's eyes were nearly swollen shut. I sent pictures via email to Dr. Steele as he'd instructed. He reminded me that swelling and bruising were expected and healing would be slow. I was grateful for his kindness and his reassurance.

Eventually David's swelling ebbed and his pain subsided, but the miracle of corrected vision that we had hoped for didn't present itself. Though David's vision improved slightly, and the images appeared closer, they remained tilted and blurred. Another burst bubble! Another dream dashed! We pushed onward, always hoping—always wishing for the next miracle.

CHAPTER 39

Wind River

In only two weeks David and I would board a plane for Colorado. It was hard to believe that nearly a year had passed since David accepted the invitation from his friend, Dr. Uldis Streips, to speak at the 2006 Wind River Conference on Prokaryotic Biology, which was celebrating its fiftieth anniversary. The conference was held near Estes Park. David was a keynote speaker. It was a distinguished honor.

When Uldis invited David to speak, David believed that he'd be entirely healed from his TBI by June 2006. I knew better. But still, I longed for any improvement. David had definitely made progress. He graduated from wheelchair to walker to cane, but his balance remained greatly impaired, and his voice, though intelligible, was scratchy. As the weeks between his eye surgery and the trip to Colorado passed, we hoped that his eye would lose its angry red, swollen appearance. It didn't. But that didn't stop David.

I knew David was nervous about the trip, but he was excited too. Our journey to Colorado would be long. It would be hard. David's bladder was still unreliable, and he'd need to use the restroom every two hours—like clockwork. This set him on edge. His ataxic hand made it difficult to release his belt and zipper, so he needed to plan his lavatory trips well in advance.

The airline attendant kindly moved our midsection seats to the front of the plane, in close proximity to the restroom. That eased some of David's anxiety, but not all of it.

We were relieved when we touched down at the Denver International Airport and saw the welcoming face of Uldis. We piled into his car and meandered an hour and a half through the winding Rocky Mountain roads until we arrived at the lodge. After David's registering and greeting old friends and my hugging my best friend Trish, David and I headed to our room. He needed to rest before dinner and his talk.

I don't remember much about the dinner. I guess I was nervous too. I sat up front for David's talk. I said I wanted to be near to assist him, but really I wanted to watch and savor each moment. I was amazed at his progress in seventeen months— from the inert body sucking life and breath from a respirator to this man who wobbled into the conference room with his cane. (He'd refused his walker.) Poised behind the lectern, he commanded the attention of his fellow scientists, their graduate students, and their postdocs.

A hush fell as the room grew dark. Before the first slide appeared, David greeted his audience. He hoped to set them at ease. He knew his appearance was startling with his crooked mouth and his puffy, post-surgery red eyes. His speech too was still raspy and gravelly, slow and exaggerated. So, after adjusting the microphone, David began, "The only complaint I've ever had from my students is that I talk too fast during my lectures. Well, I solved that problem, but I don't recommend the solution." The audience chuckled. It worked! David's joke about his condition immediately relaxed everyone, especially himself.

As the first slide appeared, David began to discuss his work: "*Actinobacillus actinomycetecomitans*: pili and adherence of an oral pathogen." I hung onto each word, though I understood nothing. David was speaking an entirely different language— the language of scientists in microbiology. In the darkness, I snuck glances at the audience. They were intent. They understood him. I sighed. The darkened room hid my tears of pride. I was bursting.

At David's last word, robust applause filled the room. I clapped the loudest and the longest. When the noise ebbed, David fielded questions. He never faltered. I was impressed, as I have been at all of his talks in England, New Zealand, Spain, Mexico, and various other places both stateside and abroad. A death-defying traumatic brain injury would not deter this scientist.

I was glad that his talk was over. Now we could relax. Well, maybe David couldn't. He had three days of meetings, workshops, poster sessions, and the talks of other scientists to attend, but I was free to hang out with Trish.

While our husbands worked, Trish and I spent nearly every minute of our days together. We enjoyed long walks in this idyllic place tucked away among the aspens more than 9,000 feet above sea level. We laughed and talked and caught up on memories as we strolled around Lily Lake. We toured the ghostly halls of the Stanley Hotel, where the story in Steven King's book *The Shining* took place, though no ghosts frolicked that day. We popped in and out of the many gift shops in the town of Estes Park. I even got a big hug from one of the local residents, a stuffed bear larger than life.

One afternoon, Trish and I kidnapped David and Uldis from their busy schedules and drove through Rocky Mountain National Park to the summit. At more than 14,000 feet above sea level, it seemed we were on top of the world.

I reflected on our good fortune as I gazed at the snow-covered peaks. I remembered how only a few weeks ago, David, in full professor regalia, tottered down the aisle on the arm of his friend, Assistant Dean Fred Loweff, amid the blue-gowned graduates at Columbia's medical and graduate student graduation ceremony.

I remembered how thrilled I was as David took his place on stage among the other capped and gowned dignitaries and how I held my breath as he hobbled to the podium to accept the Charles W. Bohmfalk Award for teaching in pre-clinical years. What an honor Columbia bestowed on him that day! That was 2006. You can imagine our surprise when David was nominated for another award in 2017! This time he was awarded the Distinguished Service Award in Basic Science. I was bursting with pride as he, once again clad in his professor cap and gown, made the trek to the podium on the arm of his colleague and long-time friend, Saul Silverstein, PhD.

I remembered too the phone call from Uldis inviting David to the Wind River Conference. A lifetime ago! I am forever grateful to Uldis for believing in his friend. I doubt Uldis realized his crucial role when, in June of 2005, he asked David to be a keynote speaker for this most important conference. I doubt he fully understood how impaired David was. Or maybe he did. But no matter—Uldis helped David realize his value in the scientific world with a TBI. Science is what David does best. He thrives on it.

I believe Columbia's honor and Uldis's faith, trust, and friendship were pivotal factors in David's recovery. Uldis took a chance on David, and they both won. David realized he could conquer anything.

We made our way down the mountain and savored our last day in this magical world, with elk roaming outside our room and hummingbirds flittering in the breeze. The meeting drew to a close. Goodbyes were shared, hugs were exchanged, and promises were made to keep in touch. I looked forward to again seeing Monique, who had done some traveling of her own while we were gone. I was eager to hear her stories and share ours with her.

CHAPTER 40

Invisible TBI

At the end of June 2006, Monique would return to Germany. I didn't want her to leave. She was like family, and I'd miss her desperately. Summer was upon us. School was nearly over, and I'd be with David full-time. I was apprehensive! I worried that I couldn't meet his many needs. Stumbling through bill paying, insurance claims, David's doctor's appointments, and fixing meals each day with no backup overwhelmed me. I'd also miss sharing my feelings with Monique. Conversely, I looked forward to regaining our private lives. I was conflicted. Fortunately, the day after we bid a sad farewell to Monique, David and I boarded a plane for San Diego—a wonderful distraction.

For the second time in two months, David was preparing a talk. He had been invited to present a synopsis of his work at a scientific symposium at the University of California at San Diego in honor of his postdoctoral mentor, Dr. Donald Helinski. Don was retiring after fifty years of scientific research. David and I and many of Don's former students and postdocs gathered at the university to honor him. Each speaker was allotted fifteen minutes at the lectern to highlight his or her work.

David's talk was scheduled directly before lunch—a time when most scientists' stomachs are rumbling, their attention ebbs, and they are eager for the session to end. David, oblivious to their needs, talked on and on and on, exceeding his time by thirty minutes. I cringed, knowing he was breaking a cardinal rule by exceeding the timer, and I knew how disgruntled these scientists would be when they could not feed their hungry bellies. I snuck glances at the audience expecting mutinous glares, but I saw only patient, accepting interest. When David finally finished to excited applause, Don Helinski was the first to acknowledge and thank him. David received many accolades, as many professors, friends, and colleagues in his field congratulated him, not only on his presentation and his delivery, but also on his determination, his motivation, and his progress through this very difficult and trying recovery.

It was refreshing to return to Southern California, where we'd spent four sun-drenched years in the mid-seventies. Our rented condo, overlooking the ocean in Cardiff-by-the-Sea, was only two blocks from the house we'd lived in when David was a postdoc at UCSD. It was as though we were transported back in time.

Liz and Ron Leavitt, who were also at the symposium, visited us. Both David and Ron worked in Don's lab in the mid-seventies. Though we'd kept up with the news through Liz's Christmas letters, we hadn't seen them in nearly thirty years.

We were saddened to learn news that Liz had not included in her yearly letters. Ron had also suffered a traumatic brain injury. He fell in his office at Brigham Young University, seriously injuring his head. Unlike David, who showed outward signs of physical disability, Ron had no visible signs of injury. This presented a new kind of suffering. Because Ron looked normal, people didn't readily realize his disability or know he'd suffered a traumatic brain injury. They didn't understand his sometimes-jumbled mind and didn't allow for his shortcomings due to his brain dysfunction. This made life in the TBI lane difficult for Ron.

Ron's fall damaged both of his frontal lobes, which affected not only his decision-making process, but also his short-term memory. That was disastrous for Ron, who is a professor of molecular biology. Liz said that, during Ron's twenty-seven years of teaching at Brigham Young University, he never used notes. He relied on his memory to deliver his lectures. Now his brain forsook him. Those once easily retainable notes became elusive, and Ron could no longer lecture.

Even I, familiar with the terrors of brain trauma, had difficulty grasping the magnitude of Ron's disability. He looked normal. No wonder he felt anxious. Realizing the deep pain and confusion that Ron suffered daily reaffirmed how grateful David and I were that David's cognitive brain remained intact. We could more easily accept his physical disabilities as we battled to overcome them.

Sure, we all looked older, but it seemed like it was only yesterday that Ron and Liz and David and I shared dinners and partied together. We enjoyed our days with Ron and Liz and hoped it would not be another thirty years before our paths crossed again.

We had more visitors during our time in Cardiff. Jared flew down from Santa Cruz to spend some quiet days with us—this place where he was born and spent his first four years. Our son's presence, the calmness of the sun hovering over the ocean, the dinner at my favorite Mexican restaurant, and coffees on the patio were exactly what we needed.

Then my mother and my brother Mark drove in from Phoenix to join us. This was the first time Mark had seen David post-trauma. His last memories of David were of a healthy, athletic, handsome, middle-aged man. I'd kept Mark informed through a plethora of emails and phone conversations, but still it was a shock for him to see the ravages of a brain trauma.

David hobbled from room to room with his four-pronged cane. He clutched a white cloth, which he obsessively dabbed at the corner of his mouth to catch the escaping saliva on his droopy lip. His right hand jiggled with a life of its own as he grasped door handles or poked light switches. He looked different from the David my brother remembered. Soon he realized that inside the shell of David's body was the same man he loved. Perhaps my emails hadn't fully conveyed the devastation of David's new life.

I was different too, though not physically. My mother, I think, saw me with new eyes—not only as a daughter, a mother, and wife, but also as caregiver, nurse, chauffeur, cheerleader, and protector as I oversaw and anticipated David's every need.

CHAPTER 41

New Normal

We headed home, leaving Cardiff-by-the-Sea behind—leaving my heart there again, but taking some happy memories with us. Nearly a year and a half had passed since it had been just David and me. It would be just us, alone again. Our days of visitor-help were over. I wasn't sure how we'd make it. I hoped that one day at a time and one step and then another would get us by. I became David's sole caregiver.

Two days a week at 9:00 a.m., a car arrived from Columbia to collect David and transport him across the George Washington Bridge to his lab for a day's work. It then returned him home at 5:00 p.m. David was in his element when he was at lab, but even the short week and abbreviated days zapped every ounce of his strength. On the days David didn't go to Columbia, I drove him to Radburn for his three one-hour therapy sessions. In addition to taking David to his many doctor appointments, I did the grocery shopping, prepared our meals, washed our clothes, paid the bills, haggled with insurance companies, and generally ran our household, which included taking out the trash—a chore that had been David's before TBI and is one I hope he will someday resume. Actually, many of those chores were David's before his trauma.

Taking on David's chores in addition to my normal ones, as

well as attending to his every need, zapped me too. I felt like an ill-equipped lifeguard in a deep, rough ocean with a struggling victim. I could barely keep my head above water, but I had to keep treading water, or we'd both drown.

When September rolled around, David returned to Columbia full-time, and I again returned to my classroom. He was not healed. I remember the doctor telling me shortly after David's last surgery that it would take at least six months for him to heal. I thought that was an unbearable amount of time. Eighteen months later, David was still severely physically disabled. Every Friday for the next seven years, David's office became his therapy gym. Allan Bateman, a preventive and rehabilitative therapist, came to David's office to work with David for two hours each session.

David still needs complete assistance on uneven surfaces, like sidewalks, streets, and grass. As his balance steadies and his confidence returns, his walking improves . . . slowly. Brain rewiring requires time. If you consider the stages a baby must master before becoming a walker—crawling, hanging onto furniture, and unsteady toddling—until he or she arrives as a secure walker, you might have a sense of what David experiences. However, for David, the process is taking vastly longer than the two years expected of a toddler to become a walking pro. I repeat, no easy task. David's brain is injured, and walking is only one hurdle he must overcome.

Thankfully his cognitive abilities were intact, which allowed him to resume his duties at lab full-time. That was his best therapy. He was picked up each day either by a car service or by a professor-friend. He was totally dependent on others in the outside world. At the end of the day, I'd meet him at the car and return him to my world—our world.

As years passed, our lives settled into new routines—our

"new normal." We went our separate ways from early morning to early evening, when we each returned home from work. I'd rush to complete my errands before arriving home, so that David and I could spend each night together. I wasn't yet comfortable leaving him alone regularly. After dinner, David would head to his makeshift office near the kitchen to work. He is always working—"doing science." It's what makes him happiest.

Though we've accepted our new life and are grateful for it, we are not yet ready to acquiesce to life in the disability lane. We peer down the TBI tunnel always searching for the light—the light that will take us closer to the way we were, to the life we enjoyed before David's traumatic brain injury. We believe it's there. We just don't know how long it will take us to reach it. But we will walk hand in hand, one step and then another, as we travel this road through life. Making it the best life we can! Together.

EPILOGUE

More than twelve years have swept by since that fateful day in January 2005 that permanently changed the directions of our lives. Gone are the days of David's racing—both foot racing and car racing. Gone too are my dreams of traveling the world together when we both retired. Our path has taken a detour, and we will amble along it to wherever it takes us—in new directions with uncharted adventures.

Much has happened in those twelve years. David's returning to work as a full-time faculty member at Columbia was crucial to his recovery. Of course, doing the same impeccable job that he always did required him to work longer. He spent much of his day and evening working. He didn't mind. He seemed to thrive on it.

David's diligent, dedicated work has produced amazing outcomes. He graduated three more graduate students with PhD degrees. Brenda Perez-Cheeks and Sarah Clock completed their work under David's guidance—much of it accomplished via hospital and home visits, which eventually evolved into email correspondence before David's return to his lab. David's last PhD student, Karin Kram, was remarkable in that she joined David's lab after his trauma—never having met David before disabilities ruled his life. She saw further than the physical. She appreciated David's intellect, his unique brain.

David notes that many people who don't know him seem intimidated by his altered appearance. I suppose it's a natural reaction. Sadly, I too plead guilty to that same behavior when I happened upon someone who looked different. I never realized how hurtful my furtive glances were. But Karin didn't allow David's distorted body to affect her decision to join his lab. Through the years after David's return to Columbia, many technicians and volunteers, including medical students, dental students, undergraduate students, and even high school summer students, as well as postdoctoral scientists, also benefited from David's scientific knowledge while they ignored his physical limitations.

David also endured the rigors of writing a National Institutes of Health (NIH) grant proposal. In these tough economic times and with the reductions in funding for scientific research, writing a fundable proposal is no easy feat. The night before the grant proposal was due, David spent the entire night completing it. I remember the night well. As he raced to the deadline, he had one request of me. He asked me to stay awake with him through the night. I did. He completed the proposal in time, and at 7:15 a.m., I, bleary-eyed, headed off to my first graders.

My sleepless night was worth it. Many months later, David and I celebrated his efforts. In this era when well-established and accomplished scientists, even those from prestigious universities, were denied funding, David was awarded an NIH grant to fund his research for five years in the amount of $1.25 million. This was the last grant proposal he'd write. Scientists are notorious for retiring late in life—working well into their seventies or eighties. That had been David's plan too, but the TBI derailed his intentions. He retired in 2013, when his grant ended. I expected to teach until then too, but New Jersey politics encouraged me to give up my passion for teaching two years sooner than I'd planned. I can't say I am entirely sad about the end of our careers. It made it possible for us to leave the New Jersey-New York area and return to the Southwest in September 2013. It allowed us to venture on to new experiences—to open new chapters in this book called life.

Before retiring in 2013, David continued to see his preventive and rehabilitation therapist, Allan Bateman. For two hours each week in David's office, they worked on David's strength and balance, which helped him walk with more ease. Although his balance has slowly improved, allowing him freedom in the house, he still requires assistance in the outside world, making him a virtual prisoner.

David's weekly visits to Dr. Lou Schimmel, his chiropractor, improved his posture, which impacted his balance. David's hunched appearance has greatly changed. He stands more erect and looks more like his pre-trauma self. David's neurologist, Dr. Michael Kailas, continued to evaluate David every three months, proclaiming him to be strong. He confessed to using David as a poster boy in his talks for medical groups. We appreciated Dr. Kailas's gentle, encouraging manner as at each visit he offered another carrot of hope.

David has endured more eye surgery to protect his cornea and to improve his eyesight, and, though his vision has improved slightly, he still lives in a blurry, tilted, and double-vision world.

David's speech is still strange. His voice is raspy and somewhat distorted, yet most people can understand him. It's not his normal voice, and it sounds like I'm living with an alien. I miss his "real" voice. Whenever I became nostalgic, I called my home phone and heard what once was. Sometimes his old voice on the message leaves me teary-eyed and longing for the days before David's brain injury. That's a slippery slope to despair. Not a place I need to go. More often, I just smile, remembering.

The ataxia in David's right hand still makes it difficult for him to type, open doors, or tie his shoes with any ease, but somehow, he gets it done. He won't accept help if he thinks he can do it himself. He never takes the easy road, and it shows. In the beginning, it'd take him thirty to sixty seconds to open the bathroom door outside my office. Forcing his hand to grasp the doorknob, then to keep it there long enough to twist and open the door was a major feat. His persistence paid off. It takes him only a few seconds to accomplish that task now.

The most radical step we took to improve David's walking was to sign up for dance lessons. I never dreamt he'd agree and he didn't disappoint me. When I broached the subject, his immediate answer was a resounding no. My talking points were ready, and I ticked them off. We were driving to Erie, so he couldn't escape my wheedling.

I explained that, when I took salsa class with my friend Vikram, I never thought I'd master the steps, but the process amazed me. As I immersed myself in learning the first step and stumbled across the dance floor, the instructor introduced the next step. As I focused on learning that step, I realized I'd actually executed the first step with ease. I internalized it, perhaps because I was focused on something else. I figured if that was subconsciously happening for me, it could also work for David. We had nothing to lose—except the rather costly price of lessons.

We had an amazing teacher. Paula Nieroda was not just a dance school instructor. She studied and analyzed David's every movement, then applied her knowledge to his sense of balance through the ballroom dances of the waltz, the Foxtrot, the swing, the cha-cha, and the tango. Imagine a dancing robot taking one painstaking step after another and hanging onto his partner for dear life, and you'd have a pretty good image of what David and I looked like in the beginning of our year and a half with Paula. By the end, when Paula left that studio, David's steps were still stilted, but we could move—note I did not say "glide"—across the dance floor. David and I both believe these lessons and Paula's sensitive, caring, and gentle, but firm, guidance improved his balance.

One of David's ventures included writing and publishing the new research data obtained by his students, postdocs, and technicians. Throughout his career he has published eighty-eight scientific papers. But the project that demanded his every waking moment when he was not at lab or working on his own research was editing a book of scientific research. The book, called *Genetic Manipulation of DNA and Protein — Examples from Current Research*, is available free online. The book presents reviews and data by twenty noted scientists from around the world. There is also a review chapter (Chapter 3) written by David that detailed the work of his lab before his retirement. The book was a daunting task. Many of the scientists, though they speak and understand English, have not mastered the art of writing in English. So David not only edited the science for accuracy, but also made certain that the writing was understandable and that it flowed.

David has always been overly busy in his life. I used to tease him and tell everyone that I had to make an appointment to speak with my own husband! He assured me it would get better. I never believed him because I know he likes it that way. Even in retirement, it's his way of coping.

I can't complain. I'm guilty of the same thing. In addition to teaching all day before I retired, I also tutored one day a week. Every Tuesday, I'd rush home to the eager face of four-year-old Eshaan. He wanted to learn Spanish. I know that sounds ludicrous, but his mother, Aparna, had found my graduate work posted on the Oregon State University website. She loved the creative lessons I presented for youngsters and asked me if I would work with her son. That was the beginning of a long, dear friendship.

Since I retired, I've filled my calendar with activities I didn't have time for while I was teaching. Before David retired and we moved to the Southwest, I became involved with two New Jersey writing groups—Pen and Prose in Nutley and The Write Group in Montclair. I was involved in a variety of writing activities at least three times a week. My favorite was the Montclair Showcase, where I'd read my work to an audience (e.g., chapters of this book as a work in progress or one of my children's picture-book manuscripts). I also enjoyed my DWT (dedicated writing time) with my writing buddies at a local coffee shop each week (where I was sitting as I wrote this epilogue).

I joined the Nutley Little Theatre, took acting classes, was an assistant stage manager for two plays, and was cast in several Reader's Theatre performances and two full-length plays. In the first play, I played the corpse. (My acting career could only go up from there!) I was excited and proud to have produced and directed my first play—a children's book that I wrote and then adapted for the stage. It was presented in October 2012. To my delight, I was also elected to and served on the board of the Nutley Little Theatre.

At least once a month, I would meet my fellow retired teachers either for breakfast and chat or for book group. Oh how the gossip flew as we caught up with news and learned about each other's lives!

In my free time (what's that?), I designed and made necklaces, bracelets, and earrings for my online jewelry site, called Diemodi Jewelry. I was often commissioned to design pieces to complement dresses for a New York City dancer. I'm also very interested in photography, and some of my photographs are displayed online and available for sale. Besides completing this book, I continue to work on several book projects that I hope to sell. Keeping busy has not been an issue in my retirement.

Without a doubt, David's traumatic brain injury has altered our lives. We can no longer hop in the car and travel to destinations unknown, as we often did. (I don't relish driving; David did.) For years following David's injury, our Friday and Saturday dinner date nights had all but disappeared, and we substituted them with a movie night at home, compliments of Netflix. (Fortunately, we have reinstated our Friday night dinner date, and we now have movie night every night. It's our way of slowing down our day.) Though most of our outings seemed to revolve around David's doctor appointments, he often attended my theater performances, and he was always in the audience when I read my work at the Montclair Library or at Barnes and Noble. He still supports me in everything I do.

With David at home now that he has retired, we spend quality time together. One of the things I love most in our retired life since we moved to the desert is that we work on my brain injury blog together, yet separately—I, in my office; David, in his.

It's not all work though. David's new recumbent trike, the Catrike 700, gets him out of the house and into the world. He loves the independence that his trike offers. David has often remarked that when he is riding, he completely forgets his varied disabilities and feels normal again. Three fifteen-mile rides each week and two more-than-sixty-minute workouts on the treadmill keep him in shape, despite his continued demand for dessert each night. I enjoy the few hours of me time in our home while David is racing through the hot, desert breeze.

I wrote this book to help others, but as any writer knows, getting a book published is more difficult than childbirth. (If you're reading this, you know that I have successfully birthed my third child—Kiersten, Jared, and now *Prisoners*.) So, while I was waiting for an agent/publisher to show interest, I felt I had to do something to help other caregivers and survivors. I had learned so much in the past twelve years, and I had to share it. So, my blog, "Surviving Traumatic Brain Injury," was born.

I've met hundreds of survivors of brain injury and caregivers, and I share their stories on my blog. But that wasn't enough. I needed to find more ways to help. I was recruited to host my own online radio show, called "Another Fork in the Road." It airs on the first and third Sundays of each month on the Brain Injury Radio Network. David works on that with me behind the scenes. He's actually done an interview with me, as have many other survivors of brain injury and caregivers. I have also written many articles about brain injury, which have been published in several online and print magazines, and I have written chapters published in books about survivors of brain injury and caregivers. I am eager to raise awareness of this silent epidemic in any way that I can.

My life in the theater has grown and expanded since we've moved to the desert. I am acting more and even joined a traveling troupe, called On the Road Productions. I've expanded my knowledge of the theater, have been stage manager for many shows, and was recently elected to the board of the Sun City Grand Drama Club. Keeping busy is my M.O. (*modus operandi*). It leaves no time to lament. It works for me. It works for David too.

Life moves on, and we don't get to pick our lane. No matter what lane we are thrust into, no matter that this disability lane is long and arduous, no matter that David's injury ripped our lives, as we knew them, apart—David and I will make the best of it and expect to enjoy every minute of it . . . together.

AFTERWORD

by David Figurski

Donna often found it difficult to write these chapters. I sometimes saw her in tears as she wrote. She intended this memoir to focus on my brain injury and what it has done to me. However, I was fascinated by another aspect of this story—it also chronicles her own experiences during this time. Because I had been "asleep" in a coma at the beginning of her ordeal, I first learned of what Donna went through during the first months of my brain injury only after she read to me the early chapters of this memoir.

The good news of my survival was not the end of Donna's ordeal. It was the beginning of a whole new life for her. Because of her love, she took care of me when I couldn't do anything. (She still takes care of me, but I'm somewhat better now.) She became a prisoner of my life as much as I became a prisoner of my disabled body. She had to observe me struggle to recover from each surgery, and she has had to accept me with numerous disabilities. I'm glad that the TBI happened to me and not to her. Still, my TBI dramatically changed Donna's life too, and now, through her account, I am fully aware of the horror of her experience.

What has my life been like after my brain injury? I'm not able to do things I want to do or readily did before. I miss the nightly walk-talks with Donna. I also miss our Friday and Saturday date nights (although we have recently restarted the

Friday date night). I hate seeing Donna's having to compensate for my disabilities, often struggling to do what I once did easily, like making repairs or lifting heavy objects. I enjoyed running fifteen to twenty miles each week. My neighbor planned for me to run a half-marathon with him the next fall. Now simply hobbling around the house takes great effort. I need to hold onto Donna to walk outside because of the slight but devastating irregularities that are essentially invisible to me. I used to work out with weights on the days I didn't run. Now, even a light bag upsets my balance, making it even more difficult to walk. I raced cars and, having won two races, was consistently competitive. I optimistically told my friend and fellow driver that I would regretfully miss a season, but it's now obvious that I'll never race again. I even sold my everyday car, since I am no longer able to drive.

I think one of the hardest parts of being a caregiver is to know when to let the survivor struggle with doing something and when not to. It's also hard for a caregiver not to take it personally when the caregiver's offer of help is refused because the survivor wants to try to do it. Donna has achieved a nice balance, but she has told me that she feels guilty letting me struggle with something even though she knows I want to do it myself. On the other hand, it's also difficult for the survivor to ask for help with something that he or she did easily before the brain injury. I've experienced this conflict myself, but I now know when to ask for help. My rule of thumb is that, if I think I can do it, I'd rather do it myself, even though it will take much longer. It's very important for my self-esteem to do it alone. When I realize I truly can't do something, only then will I ask for help.

I know people with a brain injury who appear physically

healthy but are unable to do their jobs. Some also have perceptions that don't reflect reality. I was "lucky" with my brain injury. All my disabilities are physical. My cognitive brain functions normally, and I was able to continue to direct the research of my lab and to write and publish research papers. I once lamented to my colleague and close friend, Saul Silverstein, the chair of my department at Columbia, that I wanted my life back. We both knew my wish was impossible to grant. With an impish grin, he replied, "Be thankful you can still work. Just get on with life."

Positive attitudes have been crucial to my recovery. Donna has always been supportive. She was, and still is, my personal cheerleader, my angel. In the hospital, the optimism of the doctors and nurses and especially the therapists and staff, who came to know me well, was invaluable. After I left the hospital, my advances were greatly helped by the cheerful optimism of my rehabilitative therapist, Allan Bateman, and my neurologist, Dr. Michael Kailas. The other doctors and therapists (both in New Jersey and California), the chiropractor, colleagues, students, and my lab group also were upbeat and encouraging. Our guests from Germany and my dance instructor were caring and helpful. In addition, despite my having occasional feelings of frustration and some dark moments, my keeping a sanguine attitude has been important, not only for my recovery, but also to make sure no one else is burdened by my problems.

My dreams are often dramatic and vivid. Some are good dreams, like being able to run a race. Whenever I have one of those dreams, I am comforted that I don't think of myself as being permanently disabled. Other dreams are simply inexplicable. Once I dreamed I dove into a swimming pool, but there was no water and I found myself unhurt at the bottom of a dry pool. I awoke to find myself on the floor next to my bed! Sometimes I awoke thinking that my bed was vertical and that I was staring down at the floor.

I thought I knew my body well, but becoming disabled after being healthy all my life has taught me much more about my body. One of my greatest surprises was to feel the weight of my entire body in every step. My weight hadn't been burdensome or noticeable in the past. I thought I would just have to acclimate to my body's weight again, but in a much shorter time. However, it never happened. Even walking across the room is difficult. It's clearly important for me to be strong, but what happens when I get older? Another major surprise has been my difficulty in moving after I had been sitting for a while, as I did in a seminar or at a meeting. My muscles would feel tight, and my posture was poor. I hobbled away with considerable difficulty. Eventually, as my muscles loosened, I walked better and my posture improved.

I'm happy to share my experiences about living with disabilities. Although people are usually reluctant to ask me about my life, they seem truly curious. Maybe they are worried about embarrassing me, or maybe it's they who are embarrassed. My twenty-four-year-old niece didn't know what to expect until we talked. Noticeably relieved, she proclaimed to Donna, "Uncle Dave's still in there!"

In contrast, Donna's first graders showed no hesitation in interacting with me. Every child wanted to shake my hand to experience my ataxic right arm. I told them that I can't write or draw with that hand anymore and that it can be difficult to do things, like tie my shoes. They wanted to know why my voice had been affected and why it was hard to speak. They asked me about my unsteady walking and the paralyzed half of my face.

We discussed the basics of my double vision. I tried to answer all their questions. I believe my visit was a valuable experience for them. They hopefully learned that disabled people are not different from them.

My "adventure" began while I was doing my routine morning chin-ups. I felt something pop in my head, and my focus deteriorated. Knowing that I had a problem, but not thinking that I was in danger, I went down the hall to Donna, who was getting ready for work. I had planned to stay home that day to prepare my lecture for a professor friend who was having a symposium that Saturday to honor his retirement from Wesleyan University. As I went down the hall to Donna, my right eye throbbed. I must have looked really bad because Donna was ready to call 9-1-1, which neither she nor I had ever done before.

I was describing to Donna what had happened when I suddenly felt an intense pain in my face. When I sensed fluid in my skull, I knew my brain was bleeding. To me, a brain hemorrhage meant death, and I thought then that I was going to die. Donna called 9-1-1. I was sweating profusely and fell onto the bed. Donna hurried down the stairs to unlock the door for the EMTs. As I lay on the bed in pain, I remember thinking *What a crappy way to go!* When a technician gave me oxygen, the pain lessened. Then I went into a coma.

The Sierta neurosurgeon who operated on me was clearly skilled. He saved my life. However, he was seriously deficient in interpersonal skills. How else can one explain his telling Donna at their first meeting that I would make a good organ donor? How else can one explain his informing Donna that he intended to remove me from the respirator after only one day? How else can one explain why Donna did not see him for the days following his learning that I was going to be transferred to Columbia-Presbyterian Hospital?

I believe that it's important for a physician not only to have compassion for the patient, but also to have sympathy for the worried family. Every successful applicant I interviewed for Columbia's medical school had obvious compassion and sympathy along with the expected impressive intelligence.

My coma was a strange experience. I don't know if mine was typical, but at times I heard Donna talking or reading aloud to me. I also remember my daughter and my son each holding a hand while asking me simple questions. I couldn't see them or talk to them, of course, but I could sense their excitement when I answered yes or no correctly by squeezing the appropriate hand. I remember a doctor pinching my toe. Another time, the doctor punched me really hard in the chest. In my mind, I wanted to strike back at him or her, but I was in bed, unable to see and incapable of moving.

During my coma, Donna spoke to me continuously. She always acted optimistically, even though she didn't know if any of what she was saying was getting through to me. Actually, I sometimes came close enough to consciousness that I *could* hear her. My knowing she was there and hearing her was immensely calming. I never felt that I was in danger. Donna took what eventually became a four-month leave-of-absence from a job she loved—teaching young children—so she could be at my bedside from morning until night. After I emerged from my coma, I felt that my day began only after Donna arrived in the morning. I realize now that, except for the constant presence of at least one of Avi's parents, my fellow patients had few visitors.

I didn't suddenly awake from my coma and immediately know what had happened. Instead, I needed many days to return to reality. As I neared consciousness, I became more and more aware of Donna's presence. I was able to establish that I was in a hospital. However, even when I became fully conscious, I remained confused. I was convinced that I was receiving state-of-the-art care in a hospital for race drivers! I worried about the parking fee for a car I imagined I drove to the hospital. Another time, I felt panicky because I thought I was there by mistake.

The following must have occurred not long after my transfer to Radburn. The trach had been removed because I could speak, but even though I was no longer in a coma, I was largely unaware. I can remember voices, but not images. My seven-year-old granddaughter, Kaya, annoyed that her mother, Kiersten, and her grandmother were planning to get nose beads without her, asked, "Grandpa, would you rather have your nose pierced or an aneurysm?" As I lay in bed, I answered, "An aneurysm." I don't think Kaya will ever get her nose pierced! I also remember hearing my therapists at my therapy sessions, but I recall no images of them. I only remember blackness.

After awakening from my coma, I often showed irritation, probably from frustration. Donna listened politely. At one point, Avi's exasperated father told me to stop the complaining because I was fortunate to have Donna visit me every day. I listened and tacitly agreed because I had come to the same realization shortly before. I had already planned to change my interactions with Donna. I wanted to show my gratitude for her presence. She looked out for me. She knew if a nurse made an error in my care. She made sure my wheelchair was first in line for all my therapy sessions, which she then watched intently. She tended to my comfort, making sure that my pillow was fluffed and that I was tucked in. She massaged my legs each night. Now she doesn't need to do all that, but she becomes excited by any subtle improvement.

After three months, the insurance company decided that I had been hospitalized long enough, so I was discharged. Donna knew that I wasn't ready and that I needed more time. She was right to feel anxious because I became a burden to her in many ways. On more than one occasion, Donna woke me from a deep sleep as I "screamed" in a muffled voice and punched at the air. I had been dreaming that I was being attacked, and I was trying to defend myself. I was terrified that I would hit Donna in my sleep. Understandably, she often slept with a pillow over her.

I was unable to stand when I left the hospital. Donna pushed me in a wheelchair everywhere I went. I remember practicing at home to stand in a corner (so I had the walls to minimize a fall). My goal was to stand for forty-five seconds. I often fell in the beginning, but eventually I succeeded. Then I set a longer time as the new goal. I remember the elation I felt when I stood alone and away from a corner for the first time without holding onto something for support. It happened eight months after my brain hemorrhage. I thought that standing unaided meant I would soon be able to walk unaided. Unfortunately, I was wrong.

I was astonished to hear the Columbia neurosurgeon tell me in his office that some of his patients still felt they were improving after five years. Five years! The neurosurgeon meant his statement to be encouraging, but I thought that a long recovery timeframe didn't apply to me. Now I'm in my thirteenth year, and I still have a long way to go.

Depression is common with TBI patients, and I suspected a problem in the first year. My neurologist, Dr. Kailas, prescribed a mild sedative as a sleeping aid. I was having difficulty falling asleep because I was afraid I'd never awaken. About a half year after I left Radburn, I met with the psychiatrist in the neurology ward. She assured me that TBI patients often become depressed after they realize that recovery will probably be less than 100% and that it may take a long time. Fortunately, after we talked, she concluded that I didn't need drugs or therapy.

Fourteen months after my TBI, I returned to work in my lab, first as a volunteer, then as a full-time member of the faculty again. The people in my lab group had continued to work hard in my absence. (I am grateful to the three colleagues who oversaw my lab group's projects.) I feel pleased that, since returning to work, I wrote a grant proposal to continue funding for my research, and I was later awarded a five-year research grant from the National Institutes of Health. I graduated three PhD students (the last of whom never knew me before my TBI), lectured, edited a book of international research, and continued to publish our work. Having lab meetings in the hospital and later in my living room helped me stay connected. My ability to continue with science and research was crucial to my life after TBI.

My self-esteem was boosted early when a professor friend invited me to give a keynote lecture at a conference he was organizing. I was eager to present the results of my lab group, but Donna was worried that I would not be understood only eighteen months after my TBI. Because I easily ran out of breath, I typed out my lecture word for word and indicated where I should breathe. The audience, having watched me walk slowly to the podium with a cane, appeared to be uncomfortable. To put them at ease, I started by commenting that the primary criticism by students of my lectures was that I spoke too fast. I noted that I had "solved" the problem, but that I didn't recommend the solution. The audience laughed and immediately relaxed.

My therapy was unconventional but effective. Allan Bateman, a preventive and rehabilitative therapist who worked with me in my office for a two-hour session every week after August 2006, eschews formulaic physical therapy. He has forty-five years of hands-on experience as a therapist, and he is a master in the gentle movements of Qigong and an expert in several martial arts. He adheres to the Eastern philosophy of medicine in addition to that of Western medicine. Allan tailors his therapy to the individual. He designed a unique program of exercises for me that emphasized balance, grace, and strength. It included movements from Qigong and exercises from ballet.

Probably the most unconventional activity I engaged in was a weekly dance lesson for more than a year. Dance lessons were Donna's idea. She had been impressed by her own salsa lessons. I immediately rejected the idea, thinking that I would only be learning steps. However, Donna persisted, and I listened. Finally, I agreed to one lesson without an obligation to continue. I quickly saw how mistaken I had been. Dancing is far more than knowing steps. At the end of my first lesson, I eagerly agreed to more lessons.

Paula Nieroda became my instructor. She is passionate about dancing, and she has won dance competitions. Paula has taught individuals and a variety of groups, including young children, and, to my good fortune, she generously shares her craft with the disabled. Attentive and compassionate, Paula worked with me and taught me dances that no one would have guessed I could do.

From Paula, I learned that dancers are amazingly well attuned to their bodies. She once drew for me a diagram of the sole of a foot. She then explained how one is able to tell if the body is positioned correctly by a slight increase in pressure on the ball of the foot, in the middle of the sole, or on the heel.

I think of her diagram often when I'm standing or walking. For a year, I felt that I had weekly therapy sessions from both Allan and Paula, each addressing my body from a different perspective.

An unexpected upside of my TBI is that I have made many new friends. Allan has become a close friend. Donna and I also became friends with Paula. One of my new friends is Harriet, a writing friend of Donna. Harriet has multiple sclerosis (MS). Once she asked me if, given the choice, I would choose my new life or if I would choose my life before the TBI. I thought the answer was obvious—life before my TBI. However, Harriet's answer to the analogous question for her surprised me. She became afflicted with MS late in a life she enjoyed. Yet she chose her current life. As devastating as MS has been for her, Harriet feels that she's a better person now than she was before she was ill.

The TBI left me with several disabilities: double vision; difficulty swallowing; lack of coordination of chewing, causing me to bite my lips or tongue several times a meal; partial paralysis of my tongue, making it difficult to form some letter sounds; a changed voice from altered vocal chords; an ataxic right arm; and less feeling in my right leg and foot. However, my greatest limitation is a severely reduced ability to balance. I can "walk" unsteadily inside a building, like in my home or in the Hammer Health Sciences Center, where my lab was located, but I need to hold on to someone (usually it's Donna) to walk outside, where it's not consistently level. Since my brain no longer automatically controls my balance the way it did, it's necessary that my brain now compensates. Unfortunately, conscious thought is too slow to correct a sudden loss of balance that can occur by stepping on a small stone or from a subtle change in slope.

Since an upright object takes far less energy to balance than one whose center of gravity is even slightly off-center, standing upright has become a major goal. However, my neck feels like it's connected to my toes with several strong rubber bands. I look down, not because I'm watching the floor before my feet, but because it's difficult to stand up straight. Several of Allan's exercises were designed to stretch my chest muscles to allow me to stand up straighter. Paula also emphasized an upright posture because good posture is crucial for proper dance form.

Often, I think I am standing upright, only to be told that I'm not. Once Paula videotaped my dancing with Donna. I thought that I was erect and looked pretty good. However, I was aghast at what I saw. My head was slightly forward. My back was not arched, but hunched. I was bent forward at the waist. Donna and Paula were pleased with the video because it showed my improvement. I only saw my distorted figure. The video did not show how I thought I looked.

At first, whenever I started to fall backward, I would lean forward to try to correct the imbalance with the weight of my head. That didn't work. Leaning forward made my hips go backward, and the weight of my hips made it worse! I learned that standing erect did, in fact, correct my imbalance. However, balancing by moving my head backward to stand up straight when I was already falling backward seemed scary and counterintuitive. It is like racing into a turn too fast. You desperately want to brake harder, but that move often causes a spin. The best action is counterintuitive—gently release the brakes and sometimes even press the throttle slightly to establish the correct geometry of the suspension. Lately, standing upright to balance my body is becoming more automatic, so my brain must be eliminating the need for conscious thought.

My difficulty in balancing, the double vision, and the ataxia in my right arm and hand have compromised my life the most. I have double vision because the hemorrhage killed one of the nerves needed to stimulate a muscle involved in the rotation of the right eyeball. Although the muscles attached to the other nerves attempt to compensate, the result is that one eye rotates more slowly than the other. Normally, the two images fuse, and the brain perceives one image. However, because my right eye is slow, my brain continually "sees" two images—hence, double vision. Worse, the images are tilted about fifteen degrees relative to each other.

The tilt is bad for my posture. The images are closer as I look up in my field of vision. Therefore, the images that are toward the top of my field of vision can be fused more easily. To fuse images that are straight ahead, I can tilt my body down and look up, a move that is counterproductive to good posture. My eye doctor, Dr. Vincent Vicci, designed lenses that moved my field of vision toward the bottom of the lenses. The new glasses forced me to keep my head up to see straight ahead.

I worry that my brain will "solve" the problem of double vision by suppressing its perception of one image. Double vision, annoying as it is, is also reassuring because I know that my brain perceives both images. Also, if the images fuse, I then have depth perception, although the resulting image is out of focus because my right eye is not as good as my left. Dr. Vicci designed lenses that place the images closer together. I also had surgery on my eye muscles to do the same. Neither of these procedures alone has solved the problem, but together they help.

Fusing the images must be repeated after every blink, but because there is no change in distance and the eyes are already in the correct position, fusion is quicker—generally in less than one second. Double vision changed the way I looked at a speaker and slides. Since fusion of the two images takes more time, my eyes no longer casually drift from the speaker to the slide and back like they did before. Now they tend to dwell only on the slides or on the speaker to keep the images fused. My face-to-face conversations are probably somewhat unnerving because, to maintain fusion of the two facial images, I tend to stare.

Ataxia is another major problem for me. I have learned to compensate for the ataxia where I can. For example, if I extend my arm and reach straight ahead, I can minimize the shaking. This movement allows me to initiate a handshake. When a person grasps my hand as I extend it, I am able to give a firm handshake. However, if I must grasp the other person's extended hand (as I did with Donna's first graders), the ataxia makes it very difficult.

I do as much as I can with my right hand, even if it takes me longer. My right hand is no longer as accurate and as quick as it was before the TBI. (As dean of the graduate students in the medical school, I once was meeting with two other deans when a fly became bothersome. I stabbed the air with my right hand. No one believed that I had snagged the fly, until I opened my hand and a stunned fly rolled onto the table!) Sometimes my left hand helps my ataxic right hand. It will grab an object and give it to the right hand.

I can no longer draw, which I had enjoyed, and now I must sign my name—slowly—with my left hand, which I found is not as good as it was pre TBI. I eat with my left hand, and I can no longer use a knife. I can't force my right to get the result I want. In fact, it gets worse. (I'm reminded of a sign I saw as a kid whenever I went to the neighborhood Mom and Pop grocery store: "The faster I go, the behinder I get.") The computer has been important for me. Though using my left hand on the whole keyboard is slow and awkward, the computer connects me to the outside world, and it allowed me to continue doing research. The ability to increase the font size also helps my vision. I once read prolifically, but now reading is a challenge. I listen to audiobooks whenever possible. I have learned that recovery requires considerable diligence and patience. To progress as quickly as I can, I treat every movement as therapy.

The TBI has defined a new life for me. It has already influenced a major decision. I never thought I would retire, but I did on September 1, 2013. Also, because of the TBI, I've met many new people and had experiences that I wouldn't have had without it. However, before the TBI, I felt I was on the leading edge of a hypothetical physical ability curve. Now I feel I'm simply grasping for the trailing edge.

After I retired, Donna and I moved to Arizona. We love it here, and weather is no longer an issue for me. Donna's life in her retirement has also given me a deeply felt purpose. She has dedicated her life to increasing people's awareness of brain injury. Donna has a popular blog titled "Surviving Traumatic Brain Injury," and twice a month she hosts an eighty-minute online radio show on the Brain Injury Radio Network. She has also published several articles on brain injury, and she has given a ninety-minute lecture to a local caregivers group. I use my skills to help Donna with her research, and I use my knowledge of science to find and interpret advances and new discoveries in brain research, including basic research, which she can then report in easy-to-understand language. Donna's purpose keeps us both working all day, every day.

Since Donna and I moved to Arizona, I met two people who have had a major impact on my life. Catherine "Cat" Brubaker accompanied Dan Zimmerman on a 5390-mile, five-month ride from the northwest corner of Washington State to the southern tip of Florida on their recumbent trikes. Cat is a multiple-TBI survivor, and Dan is a stroke survivor. They both live about an hour from me, so I've met with them a few times. Donna, who was following Cat and Dan's trip on her blog and radio show, was excited by the trike as therapy and encouraged me to get one. She put me in touch with Cat, who has since started a foundation to provide recumbent trikes for survivors of brain injury. Cat fortified Donna's contention and further motivated me to get a trike, so I did—the same model that Cat and Dan have.

The trike has changed my life. Unless Donna walked with me to help me balance outside, I was house-bound. On my initial ride, I was able to leave the house alone for the first time in nine years! Now my ride is fifteen miles, and I ride three times every week. (Another advantage to living here is that I can ride all year.) When I finish my ride, I feel I've had a good workout—as I did after running.

I am impressed by the survivors of brain injury I know and know of. (I have met some survivors, and I have read all the survivor interviews on Donna's blog and listened to their stories on Donna's radio show.) Every brain injury is different, and some survivors have worse issues than others. Life is frustrating and hard mentally and/or physically for survivors of brain injury, but they often show incredible courage and accomplish amazing feats. There is no question that a survivor of brain injury is reminded often of what he or she can no longer do, so every survivor needs a mental escape. When I'm riding my trike or working at my computer, I am able to forget that I am disabled. These times are extremely precious to me because they're my escapes.

My new life is certainly not what I once envisioned.

However, I refuse to be limited by my TBI. I've been given a second chance, and I want my new life to be important to others and fulfilling for Donna and me. It's up to me to make it happen.

before TBI (3 seconds)

after TBI (50 seconds)

David Figurski
Arizona

ACKNOWLEDGMENTS

Through the TBI years, David and I have become indebted to many people. It is impossible to list everyone, so please know that if your name is not included, it is not because we didn't appreciate your efforts. We *did*!

I wish to thank my publisher extraordinaire, Terri Leidich, for joining me on my journey, believing in me, and making it possible for me to share my story with the world. I am grateful to my brilliant editor, Olivia Swenson, for her amazing editing skills and for seeing the whole picture. She was a pleasure to work with. What a team!

Outstanding nurses and staff—Janice, Nina, Elizabeth, Marie, and Gil—not only provided expert care to David before, during, and after his first brain surgery, but they also cared for me. I remember their compassion still. They were *my* first responders. Thank you.

I am forever grateful to Saul Silverstein, PhD, former chairman of the Department of Microbiology at Columbia University and my magic man. He was there for me in my darkest hours and did more than I'll ever fully realize—but I have a good idea. Greatest of all, he made me laugh. Alice Prince, MD, had a major role. She not only set the wheels in motion for David's transfer to Columbia-Presbyterian Hospital—a move that no doubt was crucial to saving David's life—but she was also instrumental in choreographing David's care. Dan Fine,

DMD, was a comfort to me. He called a zillion times a day to inquire about David, and I knew he was only a phone call away.

The doctors, nurses, and support staff at Columbia-Presbyterian Hospital, especially Sander Connolly, MD, and David Markowitz, MD, both former students in David's medical microbiology lectures, and Nurse Melody, who called me in the middle of the night to provide updates on David's progress, deserve my highest praise.

David's graduate students, Brenda Perez-Cheeks and Azeem Siddique, and postdoctoral scientists, Valerie Weaver Grosso and Mladin Tomich, greeted me when I arrived at the New York apartment that Saul arranged for me to live in for the time that David would be a "guest" of Columbia-Presbyterian Hospital. I was happy to see their concerned faces and surprised to find a fully stocked refrigerator. They also kept David's laboratory running strong with the help of David's friends and colleagues who oversaw the work of his lab—Jonathan Dworkin, PhD, Howard Shuman, PhD, and Hamish Young, PhD. Edie Shumansky, the Microbiology Departmental Administrator, was amazingly adept at her job. She made sure that all of David's administrative duties were processed on time, despite his absence.

A huge hug goes to Sheryl Lloyd, my first grade aide, who left our class midday to hold my hand as David endured his first surgery. Just as big a hug goes to Karen Bennett, EdD, my principal at Honiss School in Dumont, who said, "Donna, don't worry about a thing at school. I will take care of everything"—and she did.

I am grateful to David's support doctors and therapist, all of whom oversaw his care (in alphabetical order): Allan Bateman, PRT (preventive and rehabilitative therapist); Marvin Fand, DDS (dentist); Michael Kailas, MD (neurologist); Lou Schimmel,

DC (chiropractor); and Vincent Vicci, OD, PA (optometrist). I can't say enough about the dedication of these men to David's progress and well-being as he strove to master his illness. We consider these highly qualified professionals to be dear friends.

A special thank you is given to dance instructor extraordinaire, Paula Nieroda, an amazing young woman who used dance to take David's therapy to a higher level.

Aides Artrese, Comfort, Richard, and Tracie, and many other members of the staff at the rehabilitation hospital and center provided solace and support to both David and me—but mostly to me, since David remained in a muddled state during most of his stay there. They spent many breaks chatting with me, making me smile, and assuring me that David would get well.

Jeff and Mike were David's physical and occupational therapists, respectively. Their love of their professions was obvious as they tested David and pushed him to his limits each day. A major highlight was that they welcomed me to cheerlead David through his sessions in the gym, even though a sign prominently displayed on the door denied entry to family members.

I am ever grateful to Judy Thau, the only person I know who truly and deeply understands the consequences of a spouse's traumatic brain injury, which David and I are living daily, because she is living it too with her husband, Steve. You are my beacon, Judy. You are my friend. And as you once wrote in an email to me, "You and I seem to be kindred spirits." Indeed we are! Sending you love across the miles. Give Steve a hug too. We will prevail!

When David returned to his lab at Columbia, two professors, Aaron Mitchell, PhD, and Vincent Racaniello, PhD, stepped up to drive him to lab three days a week—both going miles out of their way. The friendship, caring, and dedication of both these colleagues have touched the hearts of both David and me. Never can we thank them enough for helping to give David his life back.

When David was released from the hospital after three months, he was nowhere near being ready to be on his own. Thankfully, my daughter arranged for a friend of hers, Elisabeth (Betty), to live with us and care for David, allowing me to return to my classroom. Betty was soon followed by Kristin, Angela, and Monique. These young women were angels and will always be lifelong friends.

Our family and friend first responders traveled from every corner of the continent to be with David and me. David's father, Hank Figurski (now deceased), arrived with his sons and their wives, Tom and Kathy and Pat and Patrice. My cousins and their husbands, Patti and Bryce Williams and Kathy and Sam Spinelli, and their daughter Kayla held my hand and were frequent visitors. Christine Hayward and her husband Scott appeared with their cooler filled with sustenance—especially the chocolate-covered graham crackers—to bolster us through that long first night. Our close racing friends, Mike Marino and Angeli Kolhatkar, raced right over to lend their support. Two flat tires, fog, and delayed flights kept no one away. I was grateful for everyone's love and support. If David had not been in a coma, I know he would have expressed his gratitude too. And he would have eaten his share of the chocolate-covered graham cracker cookies.

When the hospital hullabaloo settled down and David returned home, my brother, John O'Donnell, came from Phoenix. He helped to make David's and my home more TBI friendly. He hung cabinets in the laundry room to hold David's extra supplies. He attached grab bars in stairways and bathrooms, and most importantly, he encouraged David to walk. John also helped me muddle through paying the bills. John and his wife, Carol, have been long-distance supporters from day one, guiding me through this maze of trauma even as they are engrossed in managing their own nightmare with their twenty-four-year-old son, who also had suffered a TBI.

My sister Suzanne McClain and I spent many late-night hours talking on the phone discussing David's progress—or the lack thereof. Her visit lent great support and offered me much needed comfort.

David and I are grateful to Jared's left-coast friends, Diana and Diego, Bill and Allie, and Rosie and Steve, who graciously offered us their homes the summer after the trauma so we could live in Santa Cruz near Jared. Theirs was an amazing gesture.

I credit David's Santa Cruz therapists—Mike, Mary Anne, and Gillian—with total dedication. But it was Terryn Davis who made David and me look forward to each session. Her creative therapy combined with her bubbly, infectious laughter made us laugh too. Her hour flew by.

Our niece, Caitlin Figurski, spent her Christmas break from college caring for David. She admitted at first the task frightened her, but soon she was laughing and telling everyone that her uncle was the same.

I am so glad that Aparna and Vikram Vasisht and their two sons, Eshaan and Krish, joined our life-journey. It's with deep gratitude that I thank them for their kindness and wholehearted support. They have become true friends.

I am grateful to my two writing groups, the Nutley Pen and Prose and the Montclair Write Group, who listened to many chapters from this book, giving their comments and offering encouragement. I remember fondly my writing buddies, Carl

Selinger, Karin Bates, and Janet DenBleyker, who, over coffee, a little chat, and a lot of writing, greatly encouraged me as I finished the final draft of this book.

David wishes to add to those already mentioned. He is immensely grateful to his former lab members, his colleagues on the faculty, the UMDNJ (now Rutgers School of Dental Medicine) group, as well as to the students, postdoctoral scientists, administrators, technicians, and staff in the Department of Microbiology & Immunology at Columbia University for making him feel welcome. David gives special thanks to Sankar Ghosh, PhD, the current department chairman, for his wholehearted support.

He is indebted to his New Jersey outpatient therapists: Julie (speech therapy), Rosalie (physical therapy), and Jody, Tracy, and Jill (occupational therapy). He greatly appreciated the interest and assistance of his early drivers, Esti and Asher Taboul, and he is thankful for the concern and care that his last driver, Eduardo Tejeda, had shown for over four years. David also wishes to thank Renee Woloshin and Jim O'Hara for their help and for their support of both him and me through the years.

David is very grateful to four people in the cycling world. Survivor of brain injury Catherine "Cat" Brubaker and stroke survivor Dan Zimmerman, David's recumbent trike friends, along with cyclist friends Dana and Bill Brown have opened a whole new world to David as they all cycle off into the sunset. David was greatly moved by all the cards and notes sent by well-wishers, some of whom he did not know personally, and for the generous assistance given by complete strangers.

I was so relieved when my daughter Kiersten and my son Jared dropped out of their lives at a moment's notice, leaving behind job, family, and school to rush to their father's bedside.

Our granddaughters, Treska and Kaya Stein, brought much joy to David as he floated toward the surface of consciousness. My son-in-law Falko Stein was unable to make the trip, but we felt his support. Though our daughter-in-law, Emily Hanlon Figurski, was not yet in our family picture, she is an uplifting presence in our lives now.

Finally, I am grateful to David, my husband and my best friend, who fought the greatest battle, grasping the merest thread of life, striving to overcome his roadblocks, and struggling relentlessly to regain his life—our lives. Although our lives are certainly altered, at least we have them to enjoy with each other each day, with hope and with love.

David, I love you "more most"! And three squeezes too.

Additional Information

Below are URLs with additional information about various people, organizations, and resources referenced through-out *Prisoners without Bars*. Please contact me at donnaodonnellfigurski@gmail.com with any questions.

1. Jared worked at the Maria Mitchell Aquarium on Nantucket. For more information, go to http://www.mariamitchell.org/visit/aquarium

2. While David was in the hospital, I worked on book reviews for my column Teacher's Pets on Smartwriters.com. Smartwriters.com is now defunct, but all the reviews can be found on my blog at https://donnaodonnellfigurski.wordpress.com/ and on my website at http://www.donnaodonnellfigurski.com/content/blogcategory/10/10/

   On my blog, go to Teacher's Pets: Book Reviews in the category section on the right sidebar.

3. David's interview, complete with photo, was published in the April/May 2006 issue of *In Vivo: The Newsletter of Columbia University Medical Center*. This issue can be accessed at https://wayback.archive-it.org/1914/20131211171147/http://www.cumc.columbia.edu/publications/in-vivo/vol5_2_april-may_06/at_large.html

4. Monique inspired me to get my upper lip frenulum pierced.

You can see Monique's and my piercings on my blog at https://donnaodonnellfigurski.wordpress.com/?s= monique+piercing

5. Post-TBI, David worked tirelessly on a book that presents data by twenty noted scientists from around the world. The book, called *Genetic Manipulation of DNA and Protein—Examples from Current Research,* is available free online at http://www. intechopen.com/books/genetic-manipulation-of-dna-and-protein-examples-from-current-research

   David wrote Chapter 3, which describes some of the work of his lab.

6. Paula Nieroda became David's and my dance instructor. She is passionate about dancing, and she has won dance competitions. She generously shares her craft with the disabled. Several videos can be seen at http://www.youtube.com/ watch?v=OEx2Q4kIf_o and http://www.youtube.com/ watch?v=F4j2UCWK1nk&playnext=1&list=PL827B4323119 F1BBE&feature=results_main

7. I have a blog called "Surviving Traumatic Brain Injury." It can be found at http://www.survivingtraumaticbraininjury.com

8. Twice a month, I host an eighty-minute online radio show, Another Fork in the Road, on the Brain Injury Radio Network, which can be accessed at http://www.blogtalkradio.com/ braininjuryradio

   An easier way to access my radio shows is to go to "On the Air! Show Menu" on my brain injury blog at https:// survivingtraumaticbraininjury.com/

You can find the shows in the category section in the right sidebar.

9. Here are links to some of the organizations I have found to be very helpful to brain injury survivors and caregivers:

Brain Injury Association of America: https://www.biausa. org/ (Most states have a chapter.)

BrainLine: https://www.brainline.org/

Hope Magazine: http://www.tbihopeandinspiration.com/ (Formerly TBI Hope and Inspiration)

Lash & Associates Publishing/Training Inc.: https://www. lapublishing.com/

The Mighty: https://themighty.com/topic/brain-injury/

(I have published articles in *BrainLine, Hope Magazine, Lash & Associates Publishing*, and *The Mighty*.)

About the Author

Donna has published with Scholastic, was a winner in the 2013 Legacies Writing Contest, and was recognized by the National Education Association for "Teacher's Pets," her review column for children's books. Donna is published in two anthologies on brain injury, "The Resilient Soul" and "Surviving Brain Injury: Stories of Strength and Inspiration," and with her writing group in three volumes, 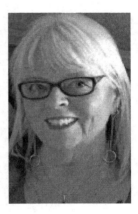 "Montclair Write Group Sampler 2014, 2016, and 2018." She is a frequent contributor to online/print journals and magazines (Hope Magazine, Lash and Associates Publishing Blog, BrainLine, The Mighty, and Disabled Magazine). She also hosts a radio show, "Another Fork in the Road," on the Brain Injury Radio Network.

Donna, a wife, mother, granny, teacher, playwright, actor, director, picture-book reviewer, photographer, and writer, states that her greatest accomplishment is being caregiver to her husband, David. Donna and David currently live in the desert. Learn more about Donna at her website: Donna O'Donnell Figurski—Author, and her blogs: Surviving Traumatic Brain Injury and Donna O'Donnell Figurski's Blog, or follow her on Facebook, Twitter, LinkedIn, and Pinterest.